due
Consideration

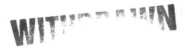

due Consideration

Controversy in the Age of Medical Miracles

Arthur Caplan

Center for Bioethics
University of Pennsylvania

JOHN WILEY & SONS, INC.

New York • Chichester • Weinheim • Brisbane • Singapore • Toronto

ACQUISITIONS EDITOR   David Harris
MARKETING MANAGERS   Catherine Beckham, Lisa Suarez
SENIOR PRODUCTION EDITOR   Jeanie Berke
DESIGNER   Harry Nolan
COVER PHOTOGRAPH: LAMB'S HEAD: Jeremy Walker © Tony Stone Images
COVER PHOTOGRAPH: HUMAN BODY: Scott Camazine/Photo Researchers

This book was set in 11/13 New Baskerville by Westchester Book Composition and printed and bound by Quinn Woodbine.
The cover was printed by Phoenix Color Corp.

This book is printed on acid-free paper. ∞

The paper in this book was manufactured by a mill whose forest management programs include sustained yield harvesting of its timberlands. Sustained yield harvesting principles ensure that the number of trees cut each year does not exceed the amount of new growth.

174.2
C172d

Library of Congress Cataloging in Publication Data:

Caplan, Arthur L.
    Due consideration : controversy in the age of medical miracles /
Arthur Caplan.
        p.   cm.
    ISBN 0-471-18344-X (pbk. : alk. paper)
    1. Medical ethics.   I. Title.
R724.C338   1997
174'.2—dc21   97–29022
                                                                              CIP

Printed in the United States of America

10 9 8 7 6 5 4 3 2 1

Many of the selections in this book had their beginnings as newspaper columns. This means that they were written late at night, in a car or on a plane. It also means that somebody, usually my wife Jane, or my son Zach, was kept waiting until I could finish the darn thing. This book is a testament to their patience.

Contents

4. THE ETHICS OF RESEARCH   75

5. NEW TREATMENT / NEW CHALLENGES   111

6. RATIONING COST   137

7. MANAGED CARE   165

8. STARTING AND STOPPING CARE   187

Introduction:
Due Consideration

The best bioethics is proactive. In order for ethics to keep up with the astonishingly rapid pace of medicine and science, it is necessary for ethics to be informed about not only the latest developments but those that are coming just down the road.

That is not easy. Science moves fast and those doing the moving are not always eager to take the time to wonder where they are going. Science can be hard to understand and nowhere is it harder to follow than out on the cutting edge of research. But the biggest reason it is hard to keep pace is because scientists are wary of sharing information about what is coming down the road with ethicists or those interested in ethics for fear that ethical concerns only spell problems for scientific advance. Or, to put the point another way, being an ethicist is the easiest thing in the world because it often appears you only need to be able to utter the word "no" with an appropriately thoughtful look on your face.

It is assumed that looking ahead through the lens of ethics leads only to the identification of problems and conundrums. As they think about the societal and moral implications of changes and innovations in biomedicine, most ethicists do seem to be wearing a permanent frown.

1

If more human beings wind up living longer, this, many glum bioethicists warn, will not be a good thing because the result will be the overpopulation of a planet already struggling with a bumper crop of doddering elders. Tomorrow's medicine may make us live longer but it is not clear that it will make us live better. The more skilled biology and medicine become at rescuing imperiled lives and extending mortally threatened ones, the worse matters seem to become in terms of strains on natural resources, diversion of economic resources to health care needs, international and intergenerational conflict, and just plain old human misery. What could be good about a future in which more and more of us make it to our seventies, eighties, and nineties to greet the Alzheimer's, parkinsonism, arthritis, or stroke that our technological arrogance has in store for us?

If we map, sequence, and crack our genetic code, can anything other then cloned hordes of totalitarian dictators and mass murderers be in the cards? How long will it really be before someone is mass producing half-animal/half-human slaves or concocting all manner of ethnic and racially targeted biological weapons?

One could make a pretty fair living forecasting and bemoaning the horrors that await us if biomedicine is permitted to proceed at its current rate of success. And many ethicists do.

There is a cottage industry afoot in the United States of experts opining that strict rationing of high technology must soon become a fact of life in the economically developed nations. The residents of underdeveloped ones have the good fortune to exit more quickly and thereby avoid the hard policy choices and even harsher policy debate about who should be tossed from the collective lifeboat. Others take no comfort from the fact that if Americans, Swedes, Germans, Canadians, Norwegians, Italians, Taiwanese, and Japanese keep spending their money on their health at their present rate, the entire gross national products of these nations will quickly be devoted to nothing else but health care. Still others in ethics find themselves petrified at the prospect of human beings so greedy for more and more life that they will prove more than willing to rob the purses of their own children and grandchildren to pay for this supremely suspect indulgence.

Admittedly, these forecasts tell us some important things about the dangers that can be associated with rapid advances in biomedicine. However, they miss the mark as to where the real focus of ethical hand-wringing ought to be.

It is tempting to ground the view that the biomedical future bodes ill on the inference that the last 50 years of medical technology have proven enormously expensive as well as morally ambivalent in terms of making us more reliant on technology and more likely to use it in war. So, it seems fair to assume that the next 50 years will hold more of the same in store. But that inference may not be valid.

If, as seems likely, medicine moves to diagnosis and treatment that is based upon interventions at the molecular level rather than at treating clinical symptoms and organ failures, there is some reason to hope that the costs of biomedical progress might actually decrease. It is a very resource intensive and, thus, very expensive process to transplant a liver from a cadaver to a child whose liver is failing due to a congenital disease like biliary atresia. Pediatric liver transplants require skilled surgery, long hospitalizations, large amounts of blood, eternal immunosuppression of the recipient, and a great deal of psychosocial support and management over an extended period for the family and the child. It should prove considerably less expensive to identify someone at risk of biliary atresia during fetal development and attempt to repair the disorder by means of introducing a vector that can carry corrective genetic information to the fetal liver or through direct genetic surgery. That would be both safer and less expensive and lead to a much happier life for the patient.

Similarly, it is very expensive to institutionalize persons with chronic schizophrenia, severe depression, or severe substance abuse problems. It may well prove far less costly to treat these same persons with a combination of designer drugs, virtual reality therapy, and micropsychosurgical or biochemical repairs.

Discussions of rationing, economic disaster, genetics run amok, and of vicious intergenerational conflicts are triggered by extrapolations from existing patterns of technological development and cost in biomedicine. Those patterns are beginning to shift, however. If the diagnostic tests beginning to appear as a result of the human genome project, biomanufacturing using transgenic animals and plants, noninvasive imaging techniques such as magnetic resonance imaging and the appearance of new vaccines for chicken pox and hepatitis are any indication, medicine's future could be both increasingly cost-effective and less invasive. It will take a great amount of skill in public policy and legislation and a fair amount of luck, but we could well find ourselves confronting a future where more of us live longer while able to function at high levels of ability for the vast portion of our lives without it costing an arm and a leg.

The most vexing ethical challenges posed by tomorrow's medicine arise at a much deeper philosophical level. If we can cure mental illness by altering the chemistry or neurology of our brains, do we risk losing our sense of personal identity in the process? If disease is diagnosed and treated most effectively at the level of molecules, will any in the health care system be capable of or get paid for actually talking to a patient? Is it irresponsible to procreate or parent without having a thorough genetic physical? Can it be in a child's best interest to be born from only one parent using cloning or after both biological parents have been dead for many years? And if we learn enormous amounts about the role played by our genes in terms of our health and functioning, who will define whether short stature, baldness, albinism, deafness, hyperactivity, or aggressiveness are classified as diseases rather than merely differences and on what basis?

It is the very reductionism that is fueling the biomedical revolution which poses the greatest moral challenge we will face. We will need to decide to what extent we want to design our descendants. We will have to grapple with the notion that we can still retain our essential humanity even if we have to modify our original biological and neurochemical blueprints in the pursuit of a longer and happier life. We will come face to face with questions about the malleability and perfectibility of our species that will make the current disputes about nature versus nurture as captured in books such as the *Bell-Shaped Curve* seem merely puerile.

Is the emerging revolution in medicine one that will leave us so befuddled about who we are and why we are here that we will yearn for simpler times when babies and children died of Tay-Sachs, sickle-cell, and cystic fibrosis while adults were ravaged by cancer, diabetes, and heart disease? Hardly.

There is always a tendency to look back longingly at times gone by. History is a funny thing. It makes the personal experiences of individuals seem simpler even as it makes the collective actions of groups more complex and confusing. But the benefits of a longer life burdened by less disability, dysfunction, and impairment, and perhaps even some enhancement of certain abilities and capacities will make the past look attractive but only as past.

The greatest source of pessimism about ethics and its relationship to science is not that ethics is often cast merely in the role of arguing against whatever it is that science seeks to do, or that progress comes with both benefits and costs, but that ethics seem irrelevant. As the moral dismay that was much in evidence in the wake of the announcement that sheep and monkeys had been cloned made very clear, there is a widespread belief that technology possesses its own momentum, that what can be done will be done, and that ethics has no power to shape, modulate, or influence the speed or direction of biomedicine. This pessimism is false.

Moral concerns have greatly altered the face of biomedicine over the past decades. What once was accepted as routine in terms of withholding information from patients about their diagnosis is today a source of a lawsuit should such information not be disclosed. The kinds of research practices that were far too prevalent in dealing with human subjects in the 1940s and 1950s have been largely eliminated through the creation of new moral standards for informed consent. And technological innovations such as the artificial heart, the use of animals as sources of organs for transplantation, the use of fetal tissue from aborted fetuses for transplantation research, and research on specially created human embryos have all been delayed or halted by moral concerns.

No doubt ethical criticism often rolls off the back of the biomedical colossus. Occasionally, however, a moral point hits its mark and biomedical research slows to take stock of what it is doing and where it is going. Ethical argument does not have the force of law. Ethical argument is often difficult to hear amid the cacophony of the marketplace. But ethical argument has authority within American and Western society and if brought to bear in an intelligent and thoughtful manner, morality has and can influence the pace and direction of biomedical research.

If one accepts the idea that it is neither arrogant nor foolhardy to want to try and modify our biological constitution and the world around us in the hopes of preventing disorder, death, and disease, then biomedicine could continue doing what it has been doing for some time, making the future better. And if we think hard about the value, principles, and virtues that should guide the evolution of biomedicine, we will be well prepared to manage whatever challenges confront us.

Arthur Caplan
http://www.med.upenn.edu/bioethics

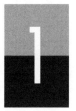

Abortion and Birth Control

Abortion, Truce?

Abortion kills. So says one popular bumper sticker in the ongoing battle over abortion. Abortion does kill. It is exacting a terrible toll on our society. Abortion is slowly killing our ability to talk to one another as fellow citizens. The cost of the abortion war is too high. It is time for a truce.

Each year in America elective abortion brings more than a million fetal lives to an end. But abortion kills more than fetuses. It has led to bombings and murder. It is the cause of the destruction of reputations and careers. Henry W. Foster, Jr., the president of Meharry Medical College in Nashville, Tennesee, and Bill Clinton's doomed nominee for Surgeon General, was one such victim.

Before he fell into the maw of the abortion war, Foster had achieved a national reputation as a leader in the field of public health. His efforts to battle the scourge of teenage pregnancy with practical programs aimed at teaching kids sexual responsibility and abstinence were recognized as being among the most effective ever undertaken in urban America. Yet, abortion left this man's work in tatters. His integrity was savaged. A man who performed abortions in circumstances where the life of a mother was in jeopardy or where a severely deformed fetus would otherwise have been born was called a "killer" and a "murderer."

The deadly effects of abortion go beyond the toll in unborn life and smashed reputations. The war over abortion has led to a complete inability to discuss the key moral issue of the day without having to listen to every crackpot, zealot, lunatic, and saliva-spewing zealot the nation houses. Abortion has deadened the editorial senses of our media that cover the debate as a battle between two extremes, those who think that the removal of a blob of tissue is a matter of complete moral indifference and those who think that it is morally justified to shoot abortion doctors in the name of God and a respect for life. It has gotten so bad that admissions of outright lying that followed on the heels of efforts to outlaw third-trimester abortions were greeted with expressions of surprise as if those writing about and reporting on the abortion debate were shocked to learn that ideologues on both sides of the issue are more than willing to play fast and loose with the facts to achieve their policy goals.

What is so startling about the way abortion is covered in the media is that almost no one holds to the views which the press features. An overwhelming majority of Americans believe that some forms of abortion are morally justified. An overwhelming majority of Americans are made morally squeamish by the existence of abortion mills and women who are having their sixth, seventh, or eighth abortions. An overwhelming majority of Americans know that there is a difference between the legal and moral status of abortion and that the morality of any particular abortion cannot be assessed without some knowledge of the circumstances. Yet, you would be hard pressed to learn any of this in a media world in which gun-toting, bull-horn blaring fruitcakes square off violently and unrelentingly against shrewish, vein-popping, tetanus-jawed nutcases.

And abortion has killed any vestige of common sense among our political leaders, who act as if there is nothing they can do except posture and preen for political advantage about an issue that ought be beyond such behavior. Whatever a woman's choice, it is one that is so difficult that to use it as a political weapon is inexcusable.

The time has come to declare a truce in a war grown intolerably strident, violent, and repugnant. Our clergy, political leaders, and business and labor communities should speak up. It is time to demand that when the subject is abortion, those who can do nothing except spew venom, hate, and intolerance will no longer have center stage in this nation. It is time to stop letting abortion claim any more political victims.

Doing Away with Late Abortions

Abortion is an issue that must be addressed on the basis of ethics not law. I say this not just because reproduction is such a deeply private and personal matter, but also because medicine and science are changing the nature and circumstances of abortion. As new forms of controlling reproduction appear, the only way to stop a woman from choosing an abortion will be to present a moral argument that she finds persuasive. If you doubt that is so, consider the hotly contested political issue of third-trimester abortions.

Throughout most of 1996, and 1997 Congress exerted a mighty effort to ban third-trimester abortions. President Clinton vetoed the ban in 1996. After Bill Clinton was reelected, the battle to ban broke out again. But, third-trimester abortions are going to disappear for reasons having nothing to do with Congress, Constitutional amendments, party platforms, politics, or state laws.

Currently available methods for detecting birth defects such as amniocentesis cannot be done until a pregnancy is well underway, around 14 to 16 weeks. Even when a test is done, it takes weeks to get a result. So some women do not find out that their fetus has a fatal disease or serious birth defect until they are entering the third-trimester of pregnancy. It is these women who make up a large number of those deciding to have the gruesome procedure that is a third-trimester abortion. This situation is about to change.

Fetal cell isolation is a new technique whereby cells from a fetus still in the womb can be withdrawn from the mother's blood without anything more invasive than a pinprick. This test can be performed early in pregnancy, around weeks nine or ten. And test results can be obtained soon thereafter. A woman who wanted to end a pregnancy because her child's brain was malformed or because the child would be born with a disabling, incurable disease could do so in the first trimester of pregnancy.

Fetal cell isolation is not yet ready for clinical use. It is only being investigated at a few medical centers on an experimental basis. But researchers are perfecting the technique and fully expect that it will replace amniocentesis and other current methods of prenatal screening for fatal or severely disabling birth defects within a few years.

When that happens, there should be far fewer reasons for women to need third-trimester abortions.

Of course the question still remains whether abortion, because of severe fetal birth defects, is ever a morally defensible choice. Surveys and polls continue to show that a majority of Americans believe that, in some circumstances, it is. What most Americans find morally disquieting about ending a pregnancy for a nonviable fetus is the timing and method used, not the reason.

Science and medicine will soon make third-trimester abortions things of the past. When that happens, those who believe that abortion due to severe fetal abnormality is immoral will have only one recourse—to put their moral case against such abortions forward with vigor, clarity, and persuasiveness.

Defrost a Fetus?

Thought about metaphysics lately? Say what? Okay, probably you haven't. But a new idea for making abortions easier for women to accept raises some tough moral questions that require thinking about metaphysics in order to answer them.

What if a woman who chose an abortion could have some of the cells of that fetus stored in such a way that a decision could be made to grow a genetically identical fetus at some time in the future? Would that be the same as killing the fetus? Believe it or not a Texas-based company is offering exactly this alternative.

Fetal reanimation is precisely what a company in Houston, Cryogenic Solutions Incorporated, wants to offer women willing to pay approximately $350. If a fetus is aborted before the eighth week of pregnancy, the company will freeze some of the fetal remains. The idea is that someday someone will figure out how to defrost some of the cells from these tissues and use them to start growing a fetus genetically identical in all respects to the one that was aborted.

I am not making this up. Some women in the Houston area have already had fetal cells frozen. The company plans to seek a patent for this idea.

The science for restarting a fetus from a fetal cell does not exist. Nor, in the view of many experts I talked with, will it ever. No one anywhere in the world has a clue how to get fetal cells growing again so that they would produce a baby. The promise being sold today of being able to try to restart the process of fetal development is exactly that—a promise but nothing more.

Science is not, however, the main obstacle to the Cryogenic Solutions Incorporated scheme for making abortion less morally controversial. The main flaw is metaphysical. It is not at all clear that growing a fetus from fetal cells obtained after an abortion is the same thing as restarting the life of that fetus.

It is hard to think of any new business venture in the history of capitalism that foundered because of a metaphysical problem with its product! But that is exactly what is wrong with the attempt by Cryogenic Solutions Incorporated to use reanimation of fetal tissue to offer women and society an alternative to the harsh realities of abortion.

If a woman decides to end a pregnancy, current technologies require that the fetus be killed. There is no getting away from this basic fact. Even if someday a scientist were able to figure out how to grow another fetus from cells preserved after an abortion, the reanimated fetus would not be the same being as the fetus that was aborted.

Two human beings that are genetically identical, that have their origins from the same embryo, are not the same person. They are what we ordinarily call twins, triplets, or quadruplets. If you grow a fetal twin, even a genetically identical copy, to replace a fetus that has been killed at six or eight weeks, whatever else you are doing you are not bringing back or restarting the same fetus. At most an extremely close copy of the original will have been created.

The identity of persons involves more than their genes. Our identity is a function of our appearance, behavior, consciousness, and genetic makeup. In addition, contrary to the vision that drives the sales pitch behind fetal reanimation, who we are is also a function of how and when we begin.

No Shortcuts

Megan Kanka, a seven-year-old Hamilton Township, New Jersey, first-grader, was strangled, raped, and killed while walking back from a friend's house. Her body was thrown into the bushes in a park near her home. The misfit who did this, Jesse Timmendequas, 33, lived across the street from the Kanka home. He had spent six years in prison for aggravated assault and attempted sexual assault of a child before moving into Megan's neighborhood.

Gary Alston was convicted in 1978 of raping a Paterson, New Jersey, woman at knifepoint. Alston abducted the woman, led her behind a building, and raped her. When two passersby approached, Alston jumped up naked and forced them away with a knife. A New Jersey judge found Alston guilty of rape, assault with intent to commit sodomy, and unlawful use of a weapon. Only the quick action of New Jersey prosecutors who knew that Alston was due for an April release despite the fact that he had been an especially bad apple in prison prevented his return to the streets.

Our legal system seems unable to deal with violent sex offenders. Medicine does no better. Treatment for the overwhelming majority of repeat offenders does not work. Frustrated legislators in some states have started calling for laws that permit repeat sexual offenders to be surgically castrated. The yelling for castration is loudest in Texas.

In 1995 the Texas senate's Health and Human Services Committee passed a bill that would have made the state the first in the nation to allow convicted sex offenders to have themselves surgically castrated. Teel Bivins, the Amarillo legislator who introduced the bill, sees nothing wrong with giving jailed sex offenders the option of having a doctor get a fee from the state to remove a prisoner's testicles. "What's more barbaric," Bivins asked, "knowing . . . that 70 percent of all the pedophiles we release are going to molest another child, or allowing . . . this voluntary treatment?"

Actually, the U.S. Department of Justice estimates the recidivism rate of untreated sex offenders as 60 percent, but no matter, Representative Bivins has a point. Why mope about the severity of surgical castration when the crimes involved are so terrible and unforgivable?

The answer is that it is dangerous to give the government the authority to use sterilization as a form of punishment. Our history is full of examples where "voluntary" sterilization for "treatment" quickly evolved into something that was neither voluntary nor treatment.

The proposed Texas law was full of language about treatment and voluntary choice. Forget it. The real sentiment behind making surgical castration legal is punishment not treatment. And saying that a certified kook residing in a prison cell who has proven capable of having sex with and then killing a seven-year-old is able to freely 'choose' castration defies even Texan standards of credulity.

Does castration work? There is some evidence from a few studies done mainly in Western Europe prior to 1980 that surgical castration strongly decreases sexual drive and aggression. The strongest claims based on this scanty evidence is that recidivism rates drop as low as 2 to 11 percent in castrated sex offenders.

But the only acceptable rate for repeat offenses with respect to violent sexual crime is zero. Who is going to feel secure knowing that the guy next door is a repeat sex offender who has merely a 2 to 11 percent chance of attacking in the neighborhood again?

The solution to dealing with violent sex offenders is to lock them up. If no one knows how to treat them, they must be kept isolated from society. Letting the government have doctors mutilate these creeps while pretending that it is at their request is to stoop to a level of negotiation and barbarity that ought to be beneath us all.

Hypocrisy and Sterilization

A mountain of phony political outrage has been built around the subject of sterilization. When Dr. Henry W. Foster, Jr., the president of Meharry Medical School who had been nominated for the office of Surgeon General, told the press that two decades ago he had performed sterilizations upon a few severely mentally impaired women, many politicians went ballistic.

Senator Orrin Hatch of Utah cried out in horror at these revelations saying he was outraged, that people should not be involuntarily sterilized. Senator Phil Gramm of Texas, Beverly LaHaye, the president of Concerned Women for America, and others on the right were soon crying quantities of crocodile tears about the horror of surgical sterilization. The politicos were soon joined by some members of the media from across the political spectrum who began gnashing their moral teeth in agony that a man capable of performing sterilizations 30 years ago could ever be considered as our Surgeon General.

The evidence that the howling over sterilization was so much hot air is readily available in the stark lack of response to the case of Cheryl Richard. Richard, 24, said that she would rather be sterilized then sent to jail. She pled guilty in a Youngstown, Ohio, court to two counts of possession of crack-cocaine pipes, one count of disorderly conduct, and one count of possession of marijuana. Municipal Court Judge Patrick V. Kerrigan sentenced her to be sterilized since "she can't seem to break out of crime and drug dependency unless some drastic measures are taken." If Ms. Richard were not forced to undergo sterilization as punishment, her petty crimes would have merited a three-month stay in jail and a $750 fine.

The judge's bizarre sentence elicited no hand-wringing by anybody. Members of Congress suddenly had no fire in their bellies concerning Ms. Richard's plight. The very same politicians and pundits who found themselves aghast at Dr. Foster's conduct more than a score of years ago were completely indifferent to the idea that a judge could sentence a woman to be sterilized for a minor crime.

Further evidence of hypocrisy rampant beyond measure about the subject of sterilization can be found in the lack of reaction, comment, or even the batting of an eyelash over the 1996 sterilization of

Cindy Wasiek. Cindy's mother worried that she might become pregnant because she was medically incapable of taking birth control pills and could be attacked and raped in her care setting. Various courts upheld the decision of the Pennsylvania Supreme Court to permit Cindy's sterilization.

The sterilization was performed. None of those who said they were consumed with ethical revulsion by sterilization were heard from. Apparently the only surgical sterilizations capable of striking moral fury in the hearts of some of our citizenry are those that were done 25 years ago by a Surgeon General wannabe who was willing to distribute condoms.

There is nothing nice about surgical sterilization. It is almost never necessary. Perhaps it should be banned altogether. But before you listen to anyone's views about the horrors of medical sterilization in the past, make them tell you their views about sterilizing Cheryl Richard and Cindy Wasiek.

The Best-kept Secret in America

Not too long ago someone I know was raped. A few days after it happened she told me about the assault. She was upset, angry, and confused. She was also betrayed by the police, medical personnel, and the pharmaceutical industry because no one offered her emergency contraception.

Women who are the victims of unwanted sexual intercourse should know that there is a pill that they can use to prevent pregnancy. If the pill were widely used it might halve the number of abortions performed in this country. Incredibly, the existence of a safe and highly effective "morning-after" pill is one of the best-kept secrets in America.

Special doses of ordinary birth control pills can be used to prevent pregnancy for as long as 72 hours after sexual intercourse has occurred. Yet, too often rape counselors, hospital emergency rooms, family doctors, student health service clinics, pharmacists, schoolteachers, pastoral counselors, and the police do not tell the victims of sexual assault about emergency contraception. This means that hundreds of thousands of women, including minor children, who are molested, attacked, or who know that a condom has broken or slipped are inexcusably left to face an unwanted pregnancy.

Emergency contraception has been around for a long time. It is standard care in Europe. The cost is minimal. Companies such as Wyeth-Ayerst and Berlex which make birth control pills have not yet sought to label and market their products as emergency contraception in this country. The FDA, which was repeatedly asked to add emergency contraception to the list of uses for birth control pills, took forever to act. Why? The only possible reasons are puritanical attitudes about sex and the politics of abortion.

There are those who actually believe that by making emergency contraception available to any women who wants it, society will encourage sexual irresponsibility. If she does it, she should pay, the troglodytes say.

Give me a break. Rape and incest have nothing to do with promiscuity. And even those who are morally indifferent about their sex lives still deserve the right to prevent an unwanted pregnancy. Withholding information about emergency contraception in the name of virtue is a sin.

The overriding reason, however, for treating emergency contraception as a state secret is abortion. The day-after-pill acts by preventing a fertilized egg from implanting. Some see this as equivalent to an abortion. Neither common sense nor biology support this view.

When the pill is taken no one knows if conception has occurred. A woman who takes the pill can hardly be said to intend an abortion. Even if there is a fertilized egg and it fails to implant, it will only be doing what huge numbers of fertilized eggs do anyway. The chance for life may begin at conception, but reproductive specialists now know that most fertilized eggs under normal circumstances do not become babies. The huge rate of spontaneous abortion makes it hard to ethically equate taking a day-after pill following a sexual assault with the surgical abortion of a fetus.

Women who are the victims of sexual assault surely deserve to know about emergency contraception. Government, health care professionals, educators, the police, the media, religious organizations, and the pharmaceutical industry should make certain that a woman who has been raped need not deal with pregnancy too.

Giving Birth in a Coma

Just over ten years ago a 19-year-old woman was involved in a terrible car accident. She was left quadriplegic and nearly comatose. After the crash she could do little more than open her eyes and emit an occasional moan. Despite her impaired condition, her parents decided that medicine ought do whatever was possible to keep her alive. Now this young woman has become the unknowing mother of a baby.

In 1996, the now 29-year-old woman was placed in a private nursing home in upstate New York. In August the nursing staff noticed something terrifying. The young woman's stomach was growing. She was pregnant. Someone had raped her. The police suspected a man who worked at the home and is known to have molested another patient.

The young woman's parents' ordeal seems beyond belief. They had to deal not only with a severely disabled daughter who cannot think or communicate but one who had been savagely raped and was pregnant. They decided to let their daughter have the baby. She was cared for by a high-risk pregnancy team at a large academic teaching hospital. The baby was born, but the family has been unwilling to talk publicly about what happened since the birth.

It is very hard to raise ethical questions about what happened in this situation. The parents have been through hell and they deserve both privacy and support as they try to cope with this tragic sequence of events. But there are important ethical questions that have to be asked about their decision.

Should the pregnancy have been continued? I have talked to a number of medical experts in obstetrics about whether a woman who has been in a coma for more than ten years can safely have a baby. They say they do not know. Pregnancy could have killed both mother and fetus. An exceedingly frail body kept alive by a feeding tube is not likely to be able to take the stress of providing sufficient support to a developing fetus.

Natural childbirth is out of the question. A fetus in these circumstances has to be surgically removed by cesarean section. That poses another risk of death for the mother.

What happens when, against the odds, a baby is born healthy

and the mother lives? I cannot even begin to imagine what it would be like to try and cope with the fact that you can never know or communicate with your mother, that she had no say at all about your birth, and that the authorities will do their best to put your father in prison for life for creating you.

Normally when persons are unable to indicate their wishes about their medical care, the place to turn is their family. For more than ten years this young woman's family has tried to act in their daughter's best interest as they saw it. Pregnancy changes that equation. The emotional conflict in trying to weigh the life of a daughter stolen from them against the welfare of a baby who holds some promise, however faint, and however bizarre, of redemption is too much to ask anyone, even the most loving and responsible parent, to bear alone.

This pregnancy should not have proceeded without an independent review of the circumstances by a court. The circumstances were so unusual and the conflicts, risks, and dangers so numerous, that someone in addition to the parents should have taken an independent look at the facts. It is impossible to imagine a court ordering a pregnancy to end against parental wishes. But a court should make sure that parents caught in such a tragic dilemma have thought through every aspect of their decision before they take their daughter and a grandchild into completely uncharted moral waters.

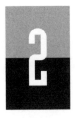

Genetics

Would You Want to Know Your Future?

What could be worse then not knowing your future? Apparently nothing given the huge numbers of people who eagerly ponder their horoscope every day or who spend money dialing the "certified" psychics who peddle their dubious skills 'round the clock on cable TV.

But would you really want to know your future if the news were bad and there was little or nothing you could do about it? If your doctor could tell you with certainty that you would be dead of a heart attack by age 45 would you really want to know? What if instead of your own future it was the medical future of your son or daughter that could be predicted? These questions, once the stuff only of novels, myths, and science fiction, are rapidly becoming real choices as two reports about genetic testing for heart disease and Alzheimer's make very clear.

In the March 15, 1996 issue of the American Heart Association's scientific journal *Circulation* a group of Australian researchers at the University of New South Wales, led by Dr. David E. L. Wilcken, report that they can identify a change in a portion of a gene that controls a chemical which regulates the body's blood pressure. This chemical, angiotensin converting enzyme, or ACE, determines how fast and how strongly blood vessels contract. Some people have a biological propensity because of the way their genes are made to make more ACE, thus leaving them at higher risk of a heart attack.

The Australian researchers looked at a group of 404 children—214 boys and 190 girls ages 6 to 13 to see if they had the genetic mutation associated with increased ACE production. They then checked the medical condition and history of the children's grandparents. When they found grandparents who had heart attacks the researchers found "a significant association between the number who had coronary events and the ACE genotype" in the children. When both grandparents had suffered heart attacks, there was a very strong link to the ACE gene marker in their grandchildren. The researchers conclude that the ACE gene mutation is a very powerful predictor of which children are at high risk of heart disease and heart attacks.

Another group of researchers at UCLA reported in the March 22 1996, issue of the *Journal of the American Medical Association* a significant correlation between the presence of a gene known as APOE and one form of Alzheimer's disease, the terrible curse that robs individuals of their memory and cognitive abilities. The UCLA group reported that in 31 subjects where older relatives had suffered from Alzheimer's, brain changes could be detected in those who had the APOE gene although no obvious signs of Alzheimer's disease were yet present.

Neither of these tests is ready for general use. But, both will be within a few years. And when they are the question that arises is what doctors should tell their patients and their families about using them.

There is little that can be done to stop the onset of Alzheimer's. Those at risk of heart disease can try to modify their diet to make it as healthy as possible, get moderate exercise, and have regular medical checkups. Of course, that is good advice for anyone to follow whether they have a genetic susceptibility to heart disease or not. In fact the same is true for many diseases that appear to have a strong genetic component: breast cancer, prostate cancer, schizophrenia, colon cancer. If you are more susceptible than others to getting these afflictions, the things you need to do are no different from what a prudent person would want to be doing anyway.

As the ability to forecast our fate by knowing something about our genes advances, we will have to decide whether knowing the future even if it cannot be altered or changed is a good thing. And, we will also have to decide whether burdening our children with the knowledge of their medical futures makes any sense if there is nothing that can be done to change or alter the risks they face.

Abe Lincoln's Genes?

Medical geneticists and advocates for patients with Marfan syndrome would like to know whether President Lincoln had the genetic disease known as Marfan syndrome. Biographers and students of our greatest president would like to know whether the depression Lincoln suffered might be linked to painful symptoms of this disease, which has its roots in genetic factors.

With the samples of Lincoln's hair, bone, and blood in the collection of the National Museum of Health and Medicine, it should be a simple matter to extract his DNA and find the answers. It would not even be expensive. But the only justification for conducting a genetic test is whether a compelling medical reason exists for doing so. And, there is none.

Even if it could be proved that Lincoln had Marfan syndrome, it would have no bearing on his presidency. Analyzing Lincoln's genes smacks more of voyeurism than of ethically responsible science.

We must be careful about genetic testing, because whether we like it or not, too much weight is often assigned to the results of such testing. There is a growing tendency to view DNA as the essence, the blueprint of humanity. People, including Lincoln, are seen more and more as the product of their genes and nothing more. Given the tendency toward placing too much weight on the role genetics plays in any life, society must be cautious about letting people explore genes—not only Lincoln's, but yours and mine.

A major moral problem in deciding whether to test Lincoln's genome is should testing be done without consent? In Honest Abe's case, the "patient" is deceased and has no survivors. There is no one to consent. Anyone who might have protested the test is long since dead. But allowing testing without consent sets a dangerous precedent.

It is strange to apply the notion of privacy and consent to the deceased. But do researchers or the public have the right to pry into Lincoln's DNA simply because neither he nor his descendants are around to invoke their right to privacy? Are we to say that anyone's body is open to examination and testing whenever a genetic test becomes available that might or might not tell us a revealing or interesting fact about their biological makeup?

Many prominent people from the past took special precautions to restrict access to their diaries, papers, and letters. Some, such as Sigmund Freud, have locked away their personal papers for 100 years. Will future Lincolns and Freuds need to embargo their mortal remains for 100 years or more to prevent unwanted genetic snooping by subsequent generations?

And when it comes right down to it, what is the real point of establishing whether or not Lincoln had Marfan? We don't have to predict from Lincoln's genotype whether he's presidential timber. He *was* presidential timber. The real questions are do we adequately understand what he did, how he behaved, what he believed—not was his genome the same as yours or mine.

Seeing Lincoln as a Marfan patient rather than as Lincoln the Great Emancipator skews our assessment of the man. People should not be reduced to a collection of chromosomes.

In the end, the genetic basis for Lincoln's behavior and leadership makes no difference. Genetic testing threatens to divert our attention from Lincoln's work, writings, thoughts, deeds, or mistakes and instead, to treat him as a jumble of DNA output. It makes more sense to encourage efforts to understand and appreciate Lincoln's legacy through his words and deeds rather than through reconstituting and analyzing his DNA. It is simply wrong to reduce a man who argued that biology ought not be destiny in American society to the product of his genes.

DNA and the Defense Department

Joseph Vlacovsky, 24, and John Mayfield, 20, were both Marine corporals stationed at Kaneohe Bay, Hawaii. Early in January of 1995 both men were ordered to report to the battalion aid station so that a small amount of their blood could be drawn and a cotton swab rubbed inside their mouths to collect saliva. They refused. They got in a whole lot of trouble because they balked at participating in the first large-scale federal program requiring genetic testing.

The Department of Defense has, since June of 1992, been collecting and storing blood samples from all active duty and reserve troops. The samples are kept in a registry maintained by the Armed Forces Institute of Pathology in Gaithersburg, Maryland. There are almost one million samples in Gaithersburg.

The rationale for the genetic registry is simple. The military wants to have a biological record of all active and reserve personnel so that there will be a way to identify bodily remains too damaged for identification by dental records or fingerprints. Genetic testing will help insure that there are fewer families left in limbo about the fate of their loved ones after a deadly battle or accident.

The way the registry works is that each soldier, sailor, or pilot's blood sample is smeared on a paper card. This card is then vacuum sealed, assigned a bar coded number, and put in a refrigerated chamber. The swab sample from the cheek is given the same code and stored in alcohol. Another blood sample is stored with the service member's military health record. If worst comes to worst, the DNA from the blood and saliva can be analyzed and matched against any cells recovered from a corpse.

The two young Marines said no one told them about any DNA testing when they enlisted. And they believed that taking and storing DNA samples violated their right to privacy. However, the main reason the two wouldn't go along with the program was their fear that genetic information about them could somehow, someday find its way into the hands of potential employers or insurers. That could mean their inability to get a job or purchase health or life insurance.

The Marines have little use for the worries of Corporals Vlacovsky and Mayfield. Both were courts-martialed. A military judge backed the two soldiers and dismissed the case. The Marines immediately appealed. A Navy–Marine Court of Military Review reinstituted their courts-martial.

It is hard not to sympathize with the military higher-ups. They want to use the latest and best techniques available to keep track of the fate of our troops. And, the Pentagon insists no one will use the armed forces DNA registry except the military. Despite these assurances, Vlacovsky and Mayfield had reason to worry. There is no federal law governing the privacy of DNA records. At any time Congress or the president could order that the specimens in the DNA bank be made available to the FBI, the CIA, health insurance companies, private businesses, local police departments, or the Medicaid program. By putting their military careers on the line the two young Marines remind us that without an absolute guarantee of privacy, compulsory DNA testing is something to fear.

Simpson Defeats Science

Lots of people are made very nervous by the rapid pace of change in science and technology. Some argue that they are so powerful, so dominant, so important in American culture that nothing, not religious, ethical, or economic concerns, can stop the forward march of scientific progress. That view is sheer nonsense. A former USC tailback and rental car shill brought science to its knees in a Los Angeles courtroom. When O. J. Simpson went free at the end of his criminal trial it was a crushing defeat for science.

Just about a week before O. J. walked out of Judge Ito's courtroom a small scientific conference was held at the other end of the nation in a small town on the Eastern Shore of Maryland. There biologists and social scientists met to discuss the question of whether there is a genetic basis for understanding violence and crime.

The consensus of the conference was that there is not. There is no such thing as a criminal chromosome or a gene responsible for making people murderers or wife beaters or liars. A number of scientists noted that not only is it meaningless to speak about a genetic basis for criminality, there is not even a basis in science for classifying people into racial groups.

The biology of human beings at the genetic level is such that the differences that we use to lump groups into categories such as white, Asian, Hispanic, Native Americans, or African Americans are not reflected in heredity. Members of the same racial and ethnic groups are as likely to have genes in common with members of other such groups as they are with members of their own. Our genetic stew is thick enough so that you have to look very hard and very carefully to even guess to what racial or ethnic group a particular person might belong. Race, one prominent biologist has told me, is nothing but a figment of our imaginations.

Some figment. Race completely defined the O. J. Simpson case. Simpson's defense team assembled a jury they thought would be favorably inclined toward their client on racial grounds. Simpson's lawyers played the race card throughout the trial. The LA police department and district attorney's office showed itself to be brimming with arrogant racists whose contempt for men of O. J.'s skin color was such that they felt comfortable lying before a rapt national audience. The incredibly accurate technology of DNA blood typing, which should have put O. J. behind bars for the rest of his life without parole, was discounted by a jury who could only see an inept and bungling police department harry a black man accused of killing two white people. The only way to interpret the O. J. trial and America's reaction to the not-guilty verdict is in terms of race.

Science says the way we use racial and ethnic terms and categories in American society is nothing but a cultural construct, a classification scheme that we impose on nature. Science and technology allow us to see that racial categories rest on trivial human differences. O. J. Simpson's criminal trial proved that, sadly, when it comes to race the nation has no interest in what science has to say.

Bah Cloning

America is hyperventilating over cloning. Before we listen to one more scenario in which unscrupulous entrepreneurs use cloning to breed spare people so we will always have an extra kidney or heart around if ours should fail, or offer to reanimate a copy of dear old Uncle Fred whose six-pack-a-day smoking habit took him from this mortal coil far too soon, lets get out our commonsense paper bags, breathe deeply, and try to catch our collective moral breath.

Don't get me wrong. Reports of successful cloning are exciting. No one knew that it would be possible to use cells taken from adult organisms and get them to work again in embryos as the Scottish research team did in producing Dolly the sheep. Success in copying monkey embryos in an Oregon primate center shows that our nearest biological kin can be cloned. These are major achievements in genetic manipulation. The living proof that it is possible to get all the genes from one creature to work when transplanted into the embryos of another certainly deserves our rapt attention. If you can get DNA from an adult sheep to fire up and make another copy of itself when put in an embryo or, split cloned primate embryos into smaller parts which then continue on to make copies of the original, it is almost a lead-pipe cinch that cloning is something that can be done in humans.

The fact that a fat and spoiled Dolly is running around in a pen in rural Scotland and a couple of monkeys are lolling about in a cage in Portland, Oregon, however, should not leave us wide awake nights wondering which ruthless totalitarian lunatic is going to send an army of specially engineered clones to attack Washington, D.C. Okay, bad example. You might fervently hope an army of clones attacks Washington. Maybe you are sure, given the huge number of indistinguishable lawyers and lobbyists ambling about the nation's capital, that the attack of the heartless clones is already well underway. Forget Washington. Substitute Mayfair, Northern Liberties, Cherry Hill or King of Prussia, or some other neighborhood, town, or locale that you love. The point is, given the state of today's cloning technology, comments about clone armies, organ farms, subhuman drones, and children miraculously brought back to life are overheated and silly.

In order to produce Dolly, Scottish scientists had to start with 300 sheep embryos. When they transferred adult genes into them the overwhelming majority of the embryos died. Others developed abnormally or produced sick and defective sheep. A similar story on a smaller scale is true of the Oregon monkey-cloning experiments.

Think of current cloning technology along the lines of the Wright brothers' first airplane flight. Many argued that human beings would never fly in a machine. The Wright brothers proved them wrong. But it took many years before the first safe, reliable, and practical aircraft was up in the air.

The same is true of cloning. The sheep in Scotland and the monkeys in Oregon represent first steps down what is a very long road. They show cloning is possible but they do not prove it is practical. The techniques used are not only not safe to try in humans, they are still not very effective or efficient for use in animals.

There is still time to control cloning technology if that is what we want to do. It will be years before today's cloning technology could reasonably be applied to human beings. If we do not want it to be, then it is up to us to engage in the moral, religious, and legal discussion that will ensure that human cloning does not happen.

The hysteria over cloning has led many experts and politicians to wonder why we should even bother to try and control its use in human beings. After all, once a technology is available its use is inevitable—isn't it? There is no stuffing the cloning genie back in its bottle. Phooey!

True no one can stop a nut from grabbing a spare embryo at an infertility clinic and transplanting adult genes into it to see if human cloning will work. But that is a long way from doing anything practical, useful, or even very interesting in terms of human cloning. If we really think that it is an offense to human dignity to have people bred by design, if it seems bizarre to let anyone create a human being just to have a place to get spare parts, or if we really do not want grieving parents trying to "restore" a lost child by making a physical copy of the child's body, we can bring such activities to a grinding halt. How? Slap stiff penalties on human cloning, let researchers know that experiments on human cloning will not be published and pull all federal and foundation support for human cloning research, and secure international agreement to treaties that prohibit any commercial return or personal profit for the creation of human clones. For all practical purposes human cloning will grind to a halt.

Do not fall for all the hype. Do not let those who learned about cloning from Woody Allen, Gregory Peck, Steven Spielberg and Michael Keaton frighten you into thinking that science and technology must inevitably be our master. Human beings can control the technologies they invent. To do so they have to use their heads not their genes.

Nature's Way?

Enjoy your Thanksgiving dinner? Got any idea where that turkey had been? What about the stuffing, tomatoes, creamed corn, pumpkin pie, and butter you ate? Are you sure they were not the products of genetic engineering?

More and more foods coming into our stores are the product of genetic engineering. Plant and animal scientists are working hard to develop strains of cows that produce more milk, pigs and steers that have leaner meat. Tomatoes, corn, and strawberries that are capable of growing in colder temperatures are already available. The humble soybean, which turns out to be an ingredient in everything you and I eat, is the object of a tremendous amount of genetic tinkering to make varieties that are more disease and pesticide resistant.

Many groups in the United States including the Pure Food Campaign, the Foundation on Economic Trends, and National Family Farm Coalition, think that food which is the result of biotechnological engineering has no place on a holiday dinner table or at any other meal. Many on the other side of the Atlantic agree. Eurocommerce, an association of more than 80 food retailers and wholesalers from 20 nations, wants legislation enacted banning the importation of any genetically engineered products.

The battle against genetically engineered foods has had an impact. Many dairies and ice cream manufacturers swear they do not use milk that comes from cows which have been genetically altered. Lots of chefs, restaurants, and health food stores are equally committed to keeping foods built by biotechnology out of their kitchens and off their shelves.

It is easy enough to get nervous when contemplating the prospect of consuming a mutant turkey or gnawing an ear of corn that contains genes dragged in from who knows where. It is hard not to cheer when your ice cream manufacturer swears that the stuff in your cone is as pure as a cow's secretions can be. Are fears of genetically engineered foods overblown?

When it comes to food there are lots of claims made about what is natural and artificial, pure or with additives, fresh or preserved, organic and nonorganic. The problem is the distinctions do not hold up. What is natural today was once very unnatural. What is fresh and pure may be nasty. And what is organic can kill you just as dead as what is inorganic.

The tangelos, avocados, and field greens beloved by many who see genetically engineered foods as unnatural are in reality the products of many decades of genetic engineering achieved through selective breeding. There is nothing remotely natural about what we call corn or strawberries. Your great-great-grandparents would not be able to identify them or almost any other foods that you and I take for granted as natural. Scientists and business have specially designed almost every fruit or vegetable you eat.

Nor is the organic, fresh, and the pure always best. Organic fruits and vegetables are fertilized with organic cow and animal manure which harbors plenty of vicious bacteria. The many recent outbreaks of E. coli and salmonella infections come from the drinking of fresh, pure unadulterated fruit juices. A little inorganic, unnatural activity can go a long way toward getting rid of some of the less friendly all-natural elements hanging around the food chain.

There is no reason to blindly accept genetically engineered foods. Consumers have every right to know what they are eating and to demand that what they eat is safe. This means taking the claims of all those who promote and advertise food, genetically engineered or not, with the help of a common inorganic substance—a grain of salt.

Perfect Christmas Trees

When I heard the disturbing news report about Christmas trees I was stuck in a long line of cars between a nursery and a small strip mall. No one would give me a break and let me get on the highway. I waited. I swore. I glanced out the window.

To my left stood a huge Styrofoam snowman listing at a precarious angle. His loss of balance did not intefere with his eagerness to persuade me I should shed some money inside his place of employ. A sign on his tilted chest urged me to take advantage of the "fire sale" on everything in the store. Snowman? Fire sale? I know times are tough but had this lopsided pitchman really thought hard about what he was saying?

To my right bobbed a nine-foot inflated Santa. He had nothing to say, but he did not have to—his appearance said it all. The left side of his head was caved in. Santa was down on his luck. He wanted me to help him by impoverishing myself in the confines of a mall that was floating his mangled body outside their premises. Still no break in the traffic. I fiddled with the radio buttons. Up popped an all news radio station.

The announcer said scientists at North Carolina State University were trying to create the perfect Christmas tree. They were scouring the United States for perfect pines, picking out the best looking ones, doing a bit of genetic analysis on the winners to make sure they were in good shape and then planning to breed them like crazy. In 30 years, one of the tree breeders drawled, everyone would have a perfect tree.

I mulled over the prospect of everyone in America gathering around perfect Christmas trees. I glanced out the window to see how my less than perfect icons of the season were receiving this news. The cranially impaired Santa and the balance-deficient snowman feigned indifference. I did not.

Until this year my wife and I always spent Christmas at her parents. There, Christmas was an extravaganza the centerpiece of which was the acquisition and mounting of the Christmas tree.

The process of getting a tree began just after Thanksgiving. A carload of people would head for a tree farm in the wilds of southern

Jersey. Shortly after getting lost, fighting would commence. By the time the tree farm was located all were in a lousy mood. The trees would be approached amid imprecations about driving inabilities and map illiteracy passing quietly from relative to relative.

The trees were never perfect. They were too bushy, too sparse, too tilted, or too wide. My mother-in-law would pick one anyway. We would tie a ribbon on it and get back to the business of getting lost.

We would return for the tree a few weeks later. It would look better but hardly perfect. Only by hiding its imperfections by carefully pushing it up against the wall could it be allowed in the house. Unfortunately, my mother-in-law has an internal plumb line that my lurching Styrofoam snowman buddy could only dream about. Not only was the tree always flawed but it was never even straight.

The tree was decorated on Christmas Eve. And then something strange happened. The flawed and tilted tree became perfect. I do not know how but it did.

I was pulled back from this reverie by high beams flashing at me. A kind soul was letting me into the traffic. I waved gratefully and then looked back in my mirror. The mashed Santa and the lurching snowman got their message across. A tree genetically engineered to perfection should never be used at Christmas.

Genetic Land Rush

Just over 100 years ago Congress gave away vast federal lands in the central part of what is now Oklahoma. Those events bear an eerie similarity to another kind of contemporary land rush—the biological race among scientists and corporations to stake claims to our genes.

What you know about the Oklahoma land rush you probably learned, as do most students of American history, from movies. Remember John Wayne, Gabby Hayes, Gene Autry, Tom Mix, Fess Parker, Gary Cooper, Clayton Moore, or whoever it was wearing a white hat and a toothy smile, steering a chuck wagon through a cloud of dust to lay claim to a swath of earth before some other equally famous Hollywood star in a black hat with a somewhat less toothy smirk got his rotten mitts on it? While no cinema stars actually rode across Oklahoma, the Hollywood version was not all that far off from the real thing. From 1891 to 1896 tens of thousands of would-be homesteaders drove their wagons into the Oklahoma territory in order to claim the best farmlands.

One hundred years later, the federal government is sponsoring a project to identify sequences of information encoded in the genes in the cells that make up our bodies. More than a billion dollars of your tax money has gone to pay for this molecular survey, the human genome project. The project has delivered. Scientists are building an impressive map of humanity's genetic code. That is why hardly a week goes by without the announcement of another genetic test for breast cancer, Alzheimer's disease, schizophrenia, or some other disease, disorder, or atypical behavior.

The opening of a new molecular world has spawned its own microscopic version of the Oklahoma land rush. Who if anyone gets to claim ownership of bits of mankind's genetic code?

One outfit with a pretty good headstart on getting its claims in early is the British pharmaceutical giant, SmithKline Beecham. The company has formed an alliance with an American company, Human Genome Sciences, to map, sequence, and patent as much of the human genome as possible. Other companies such as California-based InCyte Pharmaceuticals have saddled up their patent attorneys in an effort to lay proprietary claim to key patches of the human genome.

Some argue that it makes no sense to assign patents to sequences of genetic information simply on the basis of who finds them first. The pharmaceutical giant Merck is one of those. Merck is convinced that more money and more benefit will derive from letting all comers exploit the genetic map in order to make tests or drugs that they can then patent. Merck means it. The company is sponsoring a group at Washington University in St. Louis to find genes and put the information up on the internet for free. This has created a truly remarkable situation in which two corporate giants are engaged in a race where one is giving away what the other wishes to patent.

If government funds have been used to map and sequence the human genome, why should the fruits of that effort be turned over to the first person or company to find a particular segment? Unlike the Oklahoma land rush, society may find it unwise to award patents merely on the basis of who figures out a particular gene sequence first and gets their patent application in the fastest. It is time for Congress, the scientific establishment, and industry to undertake a more sustained examination of the role patents should play in controlling the genetic landscape. It is a lot harder to tell the good guys from the bad in the realm of genetics since unlike Gabby, Gene, and Clayton, the boys and girls heading their legal wagons out across the vast molecular prairie do not wear hats.

Patenting Genes

Does it violate God's will for the U.S. Patent and Trademark Office to allow patents on animals? According to the more than 80 prominent religious leaders who signed The Joint Appeal Against Human and Animal Patenting, it does. It is true that a visit to a patent office would persuade many that this is indeed a godforsaken place. But the reasons so many representatives of different faiths and denominations including the Southern Baptist Convention, United Methodist Church, Reformed Church in America, Reform Judaism, and the American Muslim Council raised their voices in protest go beyond the horror of experiencing a barren space filled with wastebaskets, lawyers, and other drab objects.

Some of those who signed the statement believe that allowing commercial patents on living beings, cells, or their parts is simply arrogant. Richard Ladd, executive director of the Southern Baptist Convention's Christian Life Commission, says that patenting life forms "represents the usurpation of the ownership rights of the Sovereign of the universe." Other religious leaders say they signed because patenting threatens respect for the dignity of animals and human beings by turning them into mere objects of commerce.

The statement sent a chill throughout the biotechnology industry. Large biotechnology companies like Genzyme Corporation began firing off press releases indicating that without patent protection the entire biotechnology industry will grind to a screeching halt and shortly thereafter so will America's economic future.

I must confess to a bit of amusement whenever theology manages to get the attention, even fleetingly, of commerce. But, I am afraid the case against patenting is not persuasive.

Protesting patenting in genetics in 1995 is a bit like protesting a first date between a couple who is already married and expecting a second child. The first patent on an organism was issued to the General Electric Company in 1982. The first patent on a mammal, a mouse, came in 1991. There are at least ten different rodents for which patents have been issued.

There appears to be little national angst over the fact that some biotech conglomerates have patents on a hairless mouse or an enormously obese hamster. God seems no less mighty for the fact that a couple of science wonks have grabbed a lucrative patent on a cultured human cell line. Ownership need not always lead to arrogance. The fact that I own my two collies does not make me feel like a deity. I am sometimes peeved but never arrogant when these products of genetic selection insist on going out at two in the morning.

Still, it is not clear that allowing private companies to hold patents on animals and gene sequences is sound public policy. Although the federal government has been footing the bill for most basic research in genetics for years, private companies seem to be reaping all the rewards. Shouldn't the feds try to recover a bigger piece of the biotechnology pie by retaining patents on genetic sequences discovered with grants paid for by your tax money and mine and then licensing them back to private businesses?

It is not obvious why the Deity would take offense when someone applies for a patent on a bit of DNA. But it ought to offend all of us if we foot the bill for basic research in genetics only to have private companies patent the findings and then charge us again for the use of this knowledge.

My Genes Made Me Eat It

Quit blubbering! Thus, more or less, spoke the former Surgeon General, C. Everett Koop, as he stood with a stern grimace on his bearded face next to a beaming, fit, and trim Hillary Clinton at a Washington press conference. Koop and the First Lady were there to announce his intention to carry out a war on the portly. Bill was nowhere in the vicinity, having apparently repaired to the nearest McDonald's rather than take in this latest bit of bad news.

While America's favorite doctor has enjoyed amazing success in his effort to transform cigarette smoking from a habit to a vice, he may have bit off more than he can chew in targeting tubbies for reform. He should have done better in his selection of a season for his declaration. I myself learned about his new campaign while munching on a plate of cookies at the sixth office Christmas party in a week. This is not an especially felicitous time of year to declare blubber bearers an endangered species as images of St. Nick, honeyed hams, egg nog, and sugar cookies compete for our limited attention spans.

Bad timing, however, will not confound the valiant public health Ahab from harpooning the whales among us. Koop need only wait for the traditional day after New Year's collective guilt and remorse season to commence, and his cry to liberate us from our love handles will fall on willing ears.

No, the problem Koop faces is that just a few days earlier a research team at the Rockefeller University in New York, headed by Jeffrey M. Friedman, announced the discovery of a gene responsible for obesity in humans. The researchers found that in mice, a creature that does not celebrate Christmas but which can be made to gain large amounts of weight through prolonged periods of proximate confinement during this festive time of year with bowls of M&M's Cheez-Its, and Cheez Balls, fat cells send out a chemical that tells the mouse brain when they are full. If the cells lack the right genetic message, the chemical is not made. The mouse scarfs down every bowl. The same process seems to be in place in you and me. Bad luck in nature's lottery at birth, wrong gene, no chemical, a big plate of roast beef, continued trips to the refrigerator, and the purchase of a Thighmaster follow in short order.

Dr. Koop's call for a crusade against the corpulent is certainly timely. Americans are fatter than they have ever been in their history. More than a third of us are obese, meaning we weigh more than 20 percent of what we should. The percentage of the stout jumped from 20 percent in 1970 to almost 33 percent today. Young people are much more likely to be chubby today then they were 10, 20 or 30 years ago. And, as Dr. Koop noted in launching his campaign against fat, the toll extracted by our extra pounds in terms of mortality, morbidity, and medical costs is staggering.

Koop's battle against the bulge may falter because science has just presented Americans with the excuse they have long sought for their gluttony—we cannot help it, our genes make us eat it. Forget the fact that the citizens of most other industrialized nations are not as fat as we are even though many of them too must be potential victims of the junk food lust gene. And forget the fact that when the subject is intelligence and cognitive performance, no one except ideologues looking to cut social programs or those who see Spencer Tracy and Mickey Rooney as pioneering social welfare reformers is willing to accept the idea that our fates are in our genes. If the topic is why you are a dope, it must be something that someone else failed to do for you. When the subject is your waistline, the idea that your willpower is simply a prisoner of your rampaging DNA looks mighty attractive.

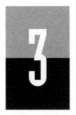

Technological Reproduction

Stolen Embryos

Ginger Canfield thinks Dr. Ricardo Asch "works for God." Ms. Canfield's reason is seven-year-old, Tessamarie Canfield.

For 12 years Ginger Canfield tried to get pregnant. It was not until Dr. Asch, the director of the Center for Reproductive Health at the University of California at Irvine, transplanted a fertilized egg into one of her fallopian tubes that she finally had the daughter she so desperately wanted.

It is one thing for a patient to think a doctor is a god. It is a very different matter for a doctor to act like a god. Dr. Asch is alleged to have done precisely that.

Records leaked to state and federal officials by courageous whistle-blowers reveal a scandal of staggering proportions at UC-Irvine. Asch apparently took eggs from one of his patients who, like Ginger Canfield, was trying to conceive, and used them to create a baby for another. No one seems to have obtained the permission of the donor or the recipient. If this charge turns out to be true, it would represent the most serious betrayal of trust in the field of infertility treatment since the birth of the first test-tube baby, Louise Brown, in England in 1978.

Making babies without consent is the most serious but not the only charge leveled against Asch and his program. The doctors at the clinic are also accused of conducting research without obtaining university approval and patient consent. Fiscal hanky-panky concerning overcharging for patient services and fertility drugs is also alleged.

The evolving scandal at the University of California-Irvine infertility program is symptomatic of a much deeper problem that has haunted the field of assisted reproduction since its inception. While the goal of assisted reproduction is a worthy one of helping infertile men and women have babies, in many parts of the country the motives of those providing the services are something less than holy.

Infertility treatment is big business in the United States. Patients pay anywhere from $6,000 to $12,000 for a single attempt at in vitro fertilization. Four, five, or more attempts are not uncommon. Asch and his associates at UC-Irvine reported earnings of $4.5 million over three years. Fifteen years ago there were fewer than 30 institutions offering test-tube baby technology in the United States. Today there are more than 250. They operate with little oversight or control.

At too many clinics the only ethic that prevails is caveat emptor—buyer beware. Can a 60-year-old woman use technology to try and have a child? Should young women be paid to take fertility drugs so their eggs can be harvested for use by others? How many embryos should be used in each attempt to make a baby? What sort of psychological screening should prospective surrogate mothers receive? What impact does a test-tube birth have on a child's self-esteem? Are there too many clinics that have not ever produced a single baby? Should the citizens of other nations be allowed to come here to find egg and sperm donors when these technologies do not exist or are scorned for religious or cultural reasons? Your guess is as good as mine, because none of these questions is covered by law, policy, or regulation. In the United States today there is more oversight of the breeding of purebred animals than there is the creation of human beings.

It would be wonderful if godlike beings provided infertility services to those who need them. The mess at UC-Irvine indicates that such is not the case. Government and the medical profession need to show less awe and more wariness of those involved in the creation of human beings.

Allwood 8

Ethical hypocrisy rose to unparalleled heights in July of 1996. No, I am not referring to the Republican National Convention, the greatest collection of wealthy white folk ever to publicly embrace economic and racial diversity in theory only. And, no, I do not refer to Bill Clinton's decision to sign a welfare reform plan that was indifferent to the welfare of children and was neither a reform nor a plan. I am talking about the pious commentary elicited by the plan of one Mandy Allwood, 31-year-old British mother of one son, living part-time with a man but not yet divorced from her husband, to bring to term eight babies.

In April of that year, Ms. Allwood began taking fertility drugs. She did so apparently unbeknownst to her on-again, off-again boyfriend, Paul Hogan. Mr. Hogan avers that he has a precise memory of the moment of passion that produced Ms. Allwood's octoplets. Baby-making, he assures all who care to know, occupied no place in his lusty thoughts. Ms. Allwood took up with Mr. Hogan despite the fact that a doctor had warned her that the drugs she used had caused her to have way too many fertile eggs and that she should not engage in sex. She was also indifferent to the fact that Mr. Hogan has taken up residence with another woman by whom he has already sired two children.

Ms. Allwood got pregnant. Really pregnant. All eight eggs were fertilized. As soon as she found out what had happened, she hired a publicist and sold the story of her miracle instant family to a trashy tabloid newspaper. The publishers of the rag promised her that if she gave birth to eight babies while giving them exclusive rights to their story, she would pocket $1 million in cash and prizes.

Sounds a little morally suspect huh? Wait, the truly hypocritical part is yet to come.

The news media, ever alert since the O. J. Simpson trial to the newsworthiness of stories being broken in supermarket tabloids, ran with the story. They ran hard. Headlines, wire stories, and editorials popped up all over the place about the gutty/goofy Brit mum who might make a cool mil and finally lasso her man if she can pop the eight tiny tykes out-of-the-oven. The problem with turning this pathetic tale into a serious news story is that those who ought to know and do better made a celebrity out of a manipulative, immoral money-grubber.

Mandy Allwood did try to deliver her fetuses. In doing so she condemned them all to a certain death.

No birth involving eight babies has ever produced a viable child. Ever. A person who would knowingly kill all her children for money does not deserve fame or publicity for her stunt. She deserves contempt. So do all the rest of those who bought into this farce.

Allwood created this mess when she had sex despite having been warned that her fertility drugs had produced too many eggs. Her doctor and pharmacist contributed to this moral mess when fertility drugs were given to a single woman who already had a son without so much as a question as to why she would want them and who she might plan to be mating with. Governments around the world continue to be complicit in fiascoes like the Mandy Allwood case by their absolute refusal to lift a pen and do anything in any way to regulate who can use reproductive technology and what rules should be followed in making babies. The media has dirty hands too. They made Allwood into exactly what she wanted—a celebrity—despite the fact that her motive in deciding to mother her babies was to win a million-dollar prize from one of the bottom-dwellers that now calls so much of the tune to which the media seem eager to dance these days.

There is a lot of blather about family values in American politics these days. Curious that when someone proposes to create a family at enormous risk solely for money so few have so little to say.

France Copes with Reproduction

The shocking scandal at the infertility program at the University of California at Irvine has left a lot of people wondering whether reproductive technologies are adequately regulated in this country. Some, including the lawyers for the three California physicians who stand accused of stealing dozens of embryos over a period of four years and using them without consent to create babies, say that the misuse of embryos is nothing more than the result of sloppy record keeping by low-ranking administrators and technicians. Many of the leaders in the field of infertility treatment say that reproductive medicine is already highly regulated and that adding more regulations would do nothing to prevent the kind of mess rocking the Irvine campus.

The desire by those in the field to dismiss the scandal at UC-Irvine as an aberration is understandable. Few people want to impose more regulation, red tape, and legal liability upon themselves. But the fact is that with the exception of a single federal law, the Wyden law requiring fertility clinics to disclose their rates of sucessfully making babies, a law that has never been enforced, there are no regulations or laws that specifically regulate the creation of children with technological assistance in the United States. American legislation says nothing about who can use infertility services, the legal status of children created by artificial insemination or in vitro fertilization, the disposition of unwanted embryos, who can donate sperm or eggs, and under what terms and what duties infertility doctors owe their patients concerning informed consent. The pathetic state of American law when it comes to watching over the powerful new ways we have to create babies becomes clear when compared with the laws that exist in France.

In July of 1994, France enacted the most comprehensive set of regulations in the world governing artificial insemination, in vitro fertilization, and other reproductive technologies. French laws are very specific and those who violate them risk both fines and imprisonment.

The French restrict access to infertility treatment to couples who can prove they have been living together for a minimum of two years. French law prohibits the insemination of single women or homosexual couples. It also bans the use of reproductive technologies to make a baby if the person who donated sperm or egg is dead.

In addition to strict eligibility criteria, French law requires those who wish to use donated sperm or eggs to consent in the presence of a judge. The law requires this be done so that if a child is born with a birth defect or some other trait or behavior the parents do not like, the parents who use donated sperm, eggs, or embryos may not reject the baby.

When embryos are frozen, both members of the couple who created them must consent in writing and both must certify annually in writing their continued desire that the embryos be kept frozen. Embryos cannot be stored for more than five years. They may be donated to another couple but to do so the recipient couple must go through a legal process similar to an adoption so there can be no battles later of who are the real parents of any child that results. Most forms of research upon human embryos are prohibited.

You may not agree with the content of the French law. I disagree with a number of the French prohibitions and restrictions on who can get access to reproductive technology and what can be done with unwanted embryos. But the point is that the French have articulated a legal and moral framework for the new world of making babies which tries to protect the interests of children created by technological means and carries real penalities and punishments for those who break the law. The United States has nothing at all. While, from the point of view of American values, the French may have gotten a lot wrong, the deplorable and inexcusable scandal at UC-Irvine ought to serve as a stimulus to public debate about the need to move in the legislative direction that the French have pioneered.

Mummy as Mommy?

Should a mummy ever be turned into a mom? In the fall of 1996 the body of a 500-year-old girl was put on display in a refrigerated case at the National Geographic Society building in Washington, D.C. No previous find was as well preserved as this one. The body was so well-preserved that it apparently triggered a bizarre request. Some researchers were interested in removing and fertilizing the mummy's eggs.

The body was found on September 8, 1995, at the 20,700-foot-high summit of Nevado Ampato in the Peruvian Andes mountains. When the girl died she was dressed in elaborately woven and colorful clothes. Archeologists think the 13- or 14-year-old was killed as part of a sacrifice which Inca priests offered to the spirits of the mountains. The spirits were thought to control rainfall crucial to the harvest. The sacrifice was seen as so important to the survival of the Inca people that families sometimes volunteered their children to the Gods.

Scientists who examined the mummified body were amazed. One scientist remarked at a press conference that he had never seen such a well-preserved set of teeth. The body was in such good condition that the tissues and bodily fluids were in nearly pristine shape. It was even possible to use modern diagnostic scanning technology to determine the exact cause of the girl's death.

She died from a blow to the head administered by a heavy club. The blow caused internal bleeding and death within a few hours. This is precisely the sort of killing associated with an Incan ritual sacrifice.

There was some uncertainty about whether or not displaying such a well-preserved body from another place and time was exploitative. But in the end public curiosity won out and the National Geographic Society put the maiden of Ampato on display in the frozen case.

Rumors flew about a very different issue. It seems that a group of scientists at a fertility clinic, upon learning that the especially well-preserved body was coming to Washington, may have made a request both to the Johns Hopkins scientists and the National Geographic Society to try and harvest some of the mummy's eggs.

Why they wanted the eggs is not clear. They may simply have

wanted to see if they still would function. Other even stranger ideas cannot be ruled out. Whatever the motives the issue of using reproductive materials from a person long since dead raises some important ethical questions.

Making mommies of mummies is immoral. Why? Because using someone's reproductive materials, their sperm or eggs, to create an embryo or fetus without their explicit consent is a violation of basic human dignity. No one should be used to reproduce without their explicit permission. To do otherwise is to remove the special status that ought to be accorded the creation of new life. Removing and fertilizing the eggs of a long since dead Inca woman is morally wrong because society has an interest in making sure that no one is forced or manipulated into reproducing without their knowledge and consent.

Buying Babies

Six-week-old Jonathan Alan Austin died on January 17, 1995, in the pediatric intensive care unit of Children's Hospital of Philadelphia. He had a fractured skull and numerous other serious injuries. How this little baby's life ended should make us all think harder about how babies are being made in America today.

The man responsible for the one-month-old boy's death is, according to Pennsylvania State Police Corporal Ralph D. Fiorenza, his father. James Alan Austin of Hanover Township, Pa., admitted to the cops that he had hit the baby on a number of occasions starting around Christmas. He was arrested on January 8 after he brought the unconscious infant to a hospital in Bethlehem, Pa. He was eventually convicted of the crime.

The fact that James Austin killed his own son is an inexcusable tragedy. The fact that James Austin basically bought his son ought to be a crime.

The 26-year-old financial analyst hired a surrogate mother, Phyllis Ann Huddleston, 29, of Lafayette, Indiana, to be inseminated with his sperm and carry the baby to term. The surrogacy was arranged by an Indianapolis outfit called the Infertility Center of America. For $30,000, Huddleston gave the boy to Austin when he was born on December 8. Austin starting beating the baby a few weeks later.

The infertility program did not seem to be especially picky about who sought their services. However, there do not appear to be any reliable screening tests that can identify potential child abusers before they get their hands on babies. Nevertheless, the question of what a 26-year-old fertile man was doing hiring a woman to have his baby cries out for some sort of answer on the part of state and federal legislators.

The ethics that seems to have governed those involved in the creation of Jonathan Alan Austin appears to be nothing more than "let the buyer beware." How can it be that more than eighteen years have passed since the appearance of the first test-tube baby, Britain's Louise Brown, and yet there are no national or international regulations or restrictions on commercial surrogacy?

In every state in this country it is illegal to sell an adult for money.

In every state in this country it is illegal for a woman to bear a child and go out into the street and auction that child to the highest bidder. However, in almost every state in this country it is entirely legal for someone to hire a woman, pay for her eggs and her uterus, and buy the baby she produces as a hired surrogate.

If the likes of James Alan Austin can simply wake up one day and decide to buy a baby, and women the likes of Phyllis Ann Huddleston can think of no better way to make a buck than to sell one, then government ought to get off its duff and get involved. Jonathan Alan Austin had no choice about who his dad would be. But society long ago ought to have made sure that no one would be able to pay somebody to make him.

Man from Mouse?

Could a mouse make a man? Well, believe it or not, some pioneering work by Professor Ralph Brinster of the University of Pennsylvania, published in the journals *Nature* and *Nature Medicine,* suggests that the answer to that question is—sort of!

Professor Brinster is the world's leading authority on the subject of spermatogenesis—how male animals produce sperm. If you are a healthy mouse or a man, there are cells in your reproductive organs, called spermatogonial stem cells, that constantly produce new sperm from puberty until the day you die.

Brinster has been doing incredibly exciting work in identifying and manipulating the cells that let male rats, mice, and men make sperm. He has shown that it is possible to take sperm-producing cells from one animal and transplant them to another and have them still function. Brinster has also frozen these cells, transplanting them later to other animals, and they still work. Most amazing of all, Brinster has successfully transplanted sperm-creating cells from rats to the reproductive organs of mice without damaging their ability to create baby rats. The implications of this pioneering research are awesome.

The ability to transplant sperm-producing cells and have them available literally forever would be of tremendous use in agriculture and veterinary medicine. Instead of freezing sperm and artificially inseminating animals as is now done, sperm-creating cells could be selected from prime stock and put into all the males in a herd. If someone wanted to preserve a rare animal's sperm, it should be possible to freeze the sperm-creating cells and reimplant them at any time, making it easier to replace nearly extinct or endangered species. But the possibilities do not end with animals. And that is where the ethical implications of Professor Brinster's research become quite interesting.

If it is possible to transplant sperm-creating cells in human males, then a man facing the prospect of infertility due to chemotherapy or radiation or occupational exposure to chemicals could have these cells removed, frozen, and put back in his body later if need be. A man who could not easily make viable sperm might accept a donation of cells from a family member or friend, or even ask a surrogate to provide his sperm-making cells. Those opposed to artificial insemination on religious grounds might find the transplantation of sperm-creating cells morally acceptable. It could even be possible to use an animal as a surrogate environment to continue a valued sperm line or to maintain a continuous source of sperm across many generations in men who volunteered or were paid to carry the gametes.

It is hard to imagine morally accepting the use of an animal as a surrogate home for human sperm cells. Someone made in this manner could well find their sense of dignity and self-worth so compromised by such an intimate tie with animal origins that it would harm them.

Thinking of a mouse or a baboon as a surrogate father may seem terrifying at best. But the moral reality is that, as with most new scientific advances, there is much good that can be done with sperm-creating cell transplants if the proper limits and directions are in place. The time to start talking about the rules of the road that ought govern the creation of life in the twenty-first century is now.

Ovary Transplants

A slew of letters have been mailed from the world-famous Genetics and I.V.F. Institute in Fairfax, Virginia, to thousands of cancer specialists all over the country. They promise hope to women facing infertility due to cancer. The letters should not have been sent.

Tens of thousands of women of child-bearing age undergo chemotherapy and radiation treatment each year for cancer. The treatment can destroy their ovaries, leaving them infertile. The doctors at the Virginia infertility clinic said that for a fee of $3,000 to $4,000 they will remove an ovary prior to cancer treatment and store it so that a portion could be retransplanted at a later date.

The most immediate problem with this form of biological insurance is that there is no evidence that it will work. The first article on ovarian transplants appeared in 1994. That study showed the technique did work. The subjects were sheep. No one has published any papers or presented any data showing that a frozen ovary can be stored successfully and then later put back and function again in a human female. So doctors treating women who are desperate to do anything to avoid the dire consequences of their cancer regimens are being asked to recruit their patients for a completely untested procedure.

The problem with efforts at recruiting large numbers of women to store their ovaries does not end with the absence of any evidence that the technique will work. Putting a transplanted ovary back into a woman who has been cured of cancer might set off a recurrence. And there is no way to know whether a baby born from eggs produced by an ovary that has been frozen and thawed will be normal.

Some might argue that if women want to spend a few thousand dollars freezing their ovaries because they fear infertility, let them. People spend equivalent sums of money all the time on equally bizarre things. Gambling casinos and state lotteries depend upon our willingness to pursue ridiculous odds. Why should the government, ethicists, or any other officious do-gooders care if someone chooses to have an ovary removed in the hope that it will work again when put back 2, 10, or 20 years later? The reason is simple.

Women with cancer who face infertility are so desperate that their consent to ovary freezing and transplant means nothing. This is especially so when one of the primary reasons for storing an ovary is to use it later to make a baby. That baby cannot consent to be a subject in what is not a cure but a desperate medical experiment.

The kind of peer review that ought to precede requests to try this sort of reproductive wizardry does not exist. The field of reproductive technology continues to resist all efforts to create any form of serious oversight. The masters of the artificial creation of life believe that the mores of the marketplace will suffice. Recruiting women for ovarian transplants proves they are wrong.

Regulating Reproductive Technologies

In 1978 on an otherwise quiet summer day, Louise Brown was born. She has grown up to be a healthy and happy young woman. There is nothing especially noteworthy about the birth of a healthy young girl in England except for the fact that the baby born on that August day started life in a way that was very different from every other person in the history of the human race. Louise Brown was conceived by means of in vitro fertilization (IVF). Her father's sperm was mixed with her mother's egg outside the body in a glass dish. The resulting embryo was transplanted back into her mother's uterus where it implanted and developed. Louise Brown was the world's first test-tube baby.

Louise's birth brought many others in its wake. More than 35,000 babies have been born using the same technique in the United States. Tens of thousands more have been born worldwide. In the late 1970s only a handful of specialized clinics in the world offered in vitro fertilization. Just in the United States today there are more than 250 clinics doing in vitro fertilization and a variety of other techniques, including the microinjection of sperm and gamete intrafallopian transfer (GIFT) to help infertile couples have babies. Over $2 billion is spent each year in the United States to treat infertility.

Louise Brown's birth brought something else in its wake—an incredible array of ethical and policy conundrums about the way medical science should be used to create and design our descendants. Hardly a month goes by without a headline concerning an issue raised by a new development in reproductive technology. Is it morally right to allow young women to sell their eggs to infertile women who cannot conceive their own in order to allow them to have a child? Is there any age at which a woman should not be allowed to try and have a baby? Is 50 too old? 55? 63? What exactly is it that makes someone a mother—a genetic tie, carrying a baby to term, bonding to the newborn infant at birth, or caring and feeding and loving a baby? What about the moral acceptability of trying to improve or enhance the traits of children by using carefully selected and screened sperm or eggs?

Moral controversy has never been far off when reproductive technology is used. Even when Louise Brown was born a moral controversy raged. Doctors, theologians, and scientists could not agree about whether it was right to even try in vitro fertlization since there was a risk that something might go wrong and the resulting child be born deformed or severely disabled.

The first test-tube baby might well have been born in the United States. But concerns about the morality of the procedure stopped early American research in its tracks. The ethical battle was so heated that it resulted in the first American attempt to create a test-tube baby ending up in a courtroom instead of a delivery room.

In the early 1970s scientist Landrum Shettles was conducting research at Columbia University Medical Center in New York City, using eggs and sperm from animals to create embryos in test tubes. He was convinced from his research and the extensive experience of animal breeders that in vitro fertlization was safe. In April 1973 he made his first attempt to fertilize a human egg outside the human body. It worked. A microscopic blob of cells could be seen under his microscope.

John and Doris Del Zio read in the newspaper about Shettles's success. They contacted him and asked that he try to help them have the baby they so desperately wanted but could not seem to conceive. On September 12, 1973, Shettles took an egg that had been surgically removed from Doris Del Zio, placed it in a dish, and added a sample of John Del Zio's sperm. A few days later, the head of the Department of Obstetrics and Gynecology where Shettles worked, Dr. Raymond Vanderwiele, who had not been asked for his permission to conduct this experiment, stormed into the lab. He destroyed whatever was in the dish. He would not, he told Shettles, risk the creation of "a monstrosity."

The Del Zios were outraged. They sued Vanderwiele and the medical center for $1.5 million. The trial, as trials are wont to do, slowly meandered its way through the New York courts. Just about the time Louise Brown was born in England late in the summer of 1978, the Del Zios were awarded $50,000 by a New York jury for psychological harm caused by the destruction of Shettles's experiment.

When Louise Brown came into this world healthy she brought one set of ethical concerns to an end. As hundreds and hundreds of other children were born over the next few years the evidence quickly mounted that being conceived in a glass dish posed no more risk for a baby then being born with the assistance of a fetal monitor or forceps.

But other issues have replaced the original ethical concern about the safety of artificial reproduction. These are no less thorny and no less contentious.

One of the most pressing issues to emerge in recent years is whether there should be any restrictions placed on who can use reproductive technologies to try and have a baby. Some infertility clinics require that those seeking their help be married. Others will take as patients single women who appear to have sufficient economic resources to raise a child. Some clinics make it clear that they will not accept homosexuals. Others specialize in helping gay people parent. Still others will take anybody, male or female, no questions asked, if they can pay.

In at least one recent instance, the lack of any rules about who can use infertility services resulted in a tragedy.

Six-week-old Jonathan Alan Austin died on January 17, 1995, in the pediatric intensive care unit of Children's Hospital of Philadelphia. He had a fractured skull and numerous other serious injuries. His father, James Alan Austin, of Hanover Township, a town just outside Bethlehem in northeast Pennsylvania, beat his son to death.

The 26-year-old unmarried financial analyst had hired a surrogate mother, Phyllis Ann Huddleston, 29, of Lafayette, Indiana, to be inseminated with his sperm and carry the baby to term. The surrogacy was arranged by a company called the Infertility Center of America. For $30,000, Huddleston gave the boy to Austin when he was born, an act she now says she deeply regrets.

Not only are there no restrictions on who can use reproductive technology to make babies, there are no restrictions on what can be done to engineer the children created by artificial means. In the small town of Escondido near San Diego, California, a sperm bank has been operating for many years with the sole purpose of making superior babies. The Repository of Germinal Choice collects sperm from men of accomplishment and, for a low fee, makes these frozen samples available to women deemed biologically worthy. The goal of this sperm bank is to produce children with special skills and abilities capable of providing the leadership needed to meet the challenges of the twenty-first century. In other words, the goal of this sperm bank is eugenics.

Eugenic goals are not so obviously in evidence in other reproductive clinics but they are there in the background. When solicitations are made for egg and sperm donors, the ads appear in college newspapers and magazines likely to be read by intelligent men and women. Some sperm banks screen their donors not only for the AIDS virus and other infectious diseases but also for their grade-point averages. Those looking to find eggs to provide menopausal women confine their search to elite universities.

Spectacular battles over the rights of those involved in using reproductive technology to make babies are all too familiar. Whether it is Mary Beth Whitehead being hired as a surrogate mother and egg donor only to change her mind about giving up the resulting baby, or the Calvert case in which an African American surrogate mother was paid to carry the embryo of an infertile married couple consisting of an Asian woman and a Caucasian man to term only to try and keep the baby, our society has sent no clear message about the custody and parental rights of egg donors, surrogates, or those who use them. Nor is it at all clear what happens when, as was true in Tennessee and New York, a couple divorces with their embryos frozen in liquid nitrogen. There are more than 30,000 embryos stored in the United States and no one knows exactly what to do with them if the people who made them divorce, die, become mentally disabled, or simply lose interest in them.

Worries about custody battles have led to some amazing ideas about where to find sperm and eggs. Some scientists have proposed taking eggs from aborted fetuses to offer to women who cannot conceive their own eggs. At least 40 requests, 25 of which have been honored, have been made during the past two years in the United States to procure sperm from men who have died suddenly, leaving their wives, fiancées, parents, or girlfriends desperate to find some way to create the man's baby. Some scientists have proposed splitting embryos through a type of cloning process to help infertile couples in need of healthy embryos.

At least one medical group at George Washington University got in trouble under circumstances eerily similar to those surrounding the work of Landrum Shettles many years earlier. The George Washington University Medical Center researchers tried to conduct a preliminary experiment to assess the possibility of splitting embryos to create cloned twins or quadrupelets. They were forced to destroy their findings when it was learned that their experiment had not been approved by the appropriate persons and committees at their medical center.

Perhaps the most exciting and most frightening research in the area of reproductive technology comes from my own university, the University of Pennsylvania. Ralph Brinster, my colleague at the Veterinary School, has succeeded in transferring genes into the cells of mice that produce sperm. Doctors and scientists have said for years that there is no reason to worry about anyone trying to genetically engineer the traits or behaviors of future generations of children because this was beyond the realm of medical possibility. However, Brinster's animal research shows at least one way in which we might decide to try and change the genetic makeup of our kids.

Oddly, one of the most common reactions to the revolution in baby making that swirls around us is despair. It seems as if the technology has bolted from the gate, and law, ethics, theology, and public policy have been left standing with their mouths open at the starting line. But this is not true. It is not too late to begin a sustained and serious societal discussion about the ethics of making babies.

The obvious value of reproductive technologies is that they enable people who could not have done so to have children. No one who has ever met a couple who has had a child after years and years of trying and failing could ever doubt the importance of these techniques to many Americans. When combined with new genetic knowledge, artificial reproduction may also allow parents to avoid having children with fatal or severely disabling disorders.

The real question is can we create a moral and legal framework for the utilization of these technologies that keeps an eye out for the best interest of the children who are created, using medical and scientific knowledge? We must make sure that the techniques are used only when they are needed for reasons that are consistent with our views about why and when people should have families and what sorts of parents and families are most likely to advance the interests of children.

Treating Infertile Men

Forget what you have heard about intergenerational warfare when it comes to paying for Social Security. The real battle between the generations, at least the male members, is about potency. Specifically do you or your dad have better sperm?

A minicontroversy is raging in American and British medical journals about whether or not men are as fertile as they once were. Some studies seem to indicate that men are no longer making as many sperm as their fathers did. Others say the quantity is about the same but today's spermatozoa just ain't what they used to be when it comes to creating babies.

While the question of whose sperm is better, yours or your father's, can certainly occupy hours of uninformed heated debate at the watercooler, local pub, or locker room, many scientists think the evidence upon which the claims for poor-mouthing the sperm of today are abysmal. There are no good records that would allow comparison of sperm counts or potency across generations. And sampling techniques vary from place to place and nation to nation.

Whatever the truth about the health of today's spermatozoa, it is true that some men are encountering problems making babies. And that raises a different question—should they be treated if they are likely to have children who also are infertile?

Some forms of male infertility are genetic. Some men simply cannot make viable sperm. Others inherit faulty genes which cause their sperm to die quickly or make it difficult for the sperm to penetrate an egg.

Advances in the understanding and identification of male infertility combined with startling progress in treatment through the microsurgical manipulation of single sperm are allowing some infertile men to father children. However, the treatment does nothing to cure the underlying cause of infertility. Male children made in this way are at a high risk of infertility too.

Surely men thinking about using the latest medical technology to treat their infertility deserve to know all the risks associated with the decision to have a child. Some parents may not wish to take the chance of passing along a genetic condition.

Intentionally creating a child with a severe congenital disability is wrong. Parents have no right to burden a child with a terrible disability. And doctors must do what they can to protect the interests of children from such a fate. However, infertility hardly ranks by itself as a problem so devastating or severe that it would be obviously wrong to create a child who is infertile.

Some argue that while it may not be immoral to knowingly create a child who faces a high risk of infertility, it is not in society's overall interest to encourage those who are infertile to reproduce. The costs involved in treating these conditions is high and the world is already an overpopulated place.

Ethical worries about the societal impact of the treatment of congenital infertility are important but none are of such moral force as to be reasons not to do so. True the pursuit of biological offspring in a crowded world is odd. Still, the value assigned to the desire to pass along one's genetic lineage or to create a biological child with another person in our culture is enormous. When sperm cannot do the job of baby making themselves, it seems right to let technology give them a boost even if the problem will be passed from father to son.

Frog Sex

When I read the headline in the *Philadelphia Inquirer* I could hardly believe my eyes. "In study, frogs reproduce in space." I read it again. Yup. Paul Recer of the Associated Press had penned a story reporting that African clawed frogs had produced tadpoles while hitching a lift on the space shuttle Endeavor. The sexual escapades of the lusty amphibians were reported in a rather staid publication otherwise not distinguished for its fascination with the prurient, the *Proceedings of the National Academy of Sciences.*

And prurient the experiment seems. Not only did the astronauts haul the frogs up into the wild blue yonder, once in orbit they injected the females with a hormone to get them to ovulate. When eggs were laid, they artificially inseminated them. Are Bill Bennett, Pat Robertson, or Phyllis Schafly aware of what is going on up there?

Wait till Jenny, Montel, Ricki, Geraldo, or one of the lesser bottom-dwelling kin who clutter daytime television get ahold of this story. The TV and print tabloid industry that has arisen to exploit the most vulnerable and pathetic saps in our midst while preaching a phony concern for their plight will eat this up. I began envisioning the promos and the headlines—NASA's latest disaster, sex on the space shuttle! Scientists say no one knows who the father is! Stowaways spend night of passion orbiting earth! etc. etc. etc.

Worse still, what will Newt, Bill and Dick Armey make of your tax money going to support the entry of a couple of truly horny leapers into the super-mile high club? Bill will surely want to spend time grilling NASA officials about how they came to spend public funds on a romantic weekend for slimy bug-eaters in a love nest so remote even a president or a congressman could not find it.

Steven D. Black of Reed College, Kenneth A. Souza of the Ames Research Center, and Richard J. Wassersug of Dalhousie University seem to have no idea what they have done in writing up their findings about the issue of this extraterrestrial fling. The scientists say there was nothing wrong with the tadpoles. Despite the absence of gravity, normal development occurred. The next step, the scientists told Recer, is to put mice or rats into space to let them indulge their most indecent thoughts. Hey, Republicans, forget the assault on the National Endowment for the Arts and the National Endowment for the Humanities. If you want a target in the culture war what about the fact that the folks at NASA are promoting bestiality above the ozone layer and writing about it in publications that children could see!

There is a point to the study of the sex life of frogs in space. By finding that gravity does not play a key role in normal embryo development scientists can see that it is chemical messages, not physical ones, that are central to how frogs and presumably you and I develop. And, more practically, should a female astronaut unknowingly enter space pregnant or become pregnant while there, these and future studies will put to rest any fears about the delivery of a child with serious medical problems as a result of fetal time in space.

So social conservatives, Bible thumpers, and cultural prudes, your fears of a craven cultural elite gutting America of values are correct. Even the space shuttle is no haven from lust and smut. If something is not done to halt this kind of thing today, who knows what men and women might be doing up there tomorrow?

Sperm from the Dead

Anthony and Maribel Baez were married in June of 1992. Two-and-a-half years later, on December 22, 1994, while visiting relatives in New York, the 29-year-old machine shop operator from Orlando, Florida, died on a street corner in the Bronx after an altercation with the police. Despite his sudden death, Maribel plans to become pregnant using her husband's sperm.

The ability to make a baby long after a man has died is the latest twist in reproductive technology. Moral and legal debate is not keeping abreast of developments with respect to making babies. It is a gap that desperately needs to be closed.

The Baez family's attorney says the police killed Baez using an illegal chokehold after he got into an argument with them. The medical examiner thinks the death is suspicious enough to label a "homicide." An investigation was launched into the conduct of the police by the district attorney.

When Anthony Baez was brought to the New York City morgue, all his wife could think about were the children that they had wanted to have. She asked the assistant medical examiner if there was any way "to save Tony's sperm." A few phone calls were made and eventually Dr. Peter Schlegel, a urologist specializing in male infertility at New York Hospital-Cornell Medical Center, was found.

Dr. Schlegel knew that it was theoretically possible to obtain sperm from a corpse. He also knew that sperm could only live for 24 hours outside the body and that he had little time left if he was going to try to get a sample from Baez's body. He drove to the morgue, performed the surgery to obtain the sperm, examined it on the spot under a microscope and, satisfied it was healthy, had it rushed to a sperm bank located in the Empire State Building where it was frozen and is now being stored.

Schlegel thought he had done the first procurement of sperm from a corpse. But, in fact, the procedure has been done more than two dozen times in medical centers around the United States, sometimes for a wife, sometimes for a fiancée, and on one occasion for a woman who had been dating a man for a long time prior to his death.

It is not clear that Dr. Schlegel or Maribel did anything wrong when they took sperm from the body of Anthony Baez. Certainly Maribel knew whether Anthony wanted children and, as his wife, she has a claim over the disposition of his body. Although what happened in this case is not morally troubling, there are some very hard questions that need to be asked about the morality of taking sperm from the dead.

Whenever a man dies should sperm retrieval be offered to his loved ones? And, while the technology is not yet here for freezing eggs, in some cases it might be possible to take an egg from a woman who has died, have it fertilized by a spouse or lover and then frozen. Many Americans routinely carry organ-donor cards. Should these include sections about postmortem donations of sperm, eggs, or embryos? And, who should have access to reproductive materials? Is a marriage license enough or is the stated intent on the part of the deceased to someday have children required? If reproductive materials are stored as has happened in the Baez case, how long should they be kept before being either used or destroyed?

The moral twists and turns involved with allowing the creation of babies after death are incredible. Still, as the Baez case makes clear, technology can help some whom death once would have robbed of the chance to create a new life to have a baby with the person they loved most. Our challenge is to design public policies to govern our new knowledge of how to make a child that allow miracles to happen with a minimum of misery.

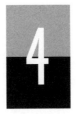

The Ethics of Research

- Ounce of Prevention
- Misconduct
- In Industry We Should Trust?
- The FDA Will Bury You!
- Labs Rats Put On a Few Ounces
- Research in an Emergency
- The Return of Thalidomide
- Acne, Accutane, and Ethics
- Give 'Em an Inch
- Betrayal of Trust
- What We Do for Animals We Should Do for People

Ounce of Prevention

Skeptical that science can produce a potboiler of a story with enough deceit and intrigue to make even the most jaded soap opera producer sit up and take notice? Consider the case of Margot O'Toole.

The O'Toole case ended after a ten year battle. A three-member government panel found no basis in O'Toole's charges of fraud in an important scientific experiment. By the time the fraud charges were resolved the careers of most of the participants involved in this mess were in a shambles and the scientific community was in an uproar.

The suspect data appeared in a paper published in a very prestigious journal, *Cell,* that included among its authors a Nobel prize-winning biologist, David Baltimore. Baltimore is indisputably one of the giants of twentieth-century American science. The lead author of the paper was a tough-minded, hardworking woman from Brazil, Theresa Imanishi-Kari. Her work, and thus, Baltimore's too, was challenged as fabricated by a newly minted young scientist, Margot O'Toole. All hell then broke loose.

Investigations were launched at the researcher's home institutions, Tufts University and MIT. No misconduct was found. Then the National Institutes of Health got involved. After another inquiry into O'Toole's charges the authors were directed to publish a minor correction. O'Toole, unmoved, insisted that the published data were wrong. She got the attention of a powerful congressman, Michigan's John Dingell, who played a key role in the politics of budget allocation for American medical research. Soon Dingell had the Secret Service and a newly formed agency, the Office of Scientific Integrity, swarming over Imanishi-Kari's lab records. But she and Baltimore stuck to their guns, insisting that nothing was amiss.

As a result of the charges and the investigations, Baltimore was forced to resign his position as president of Rockefeller University as some of the faculty at this world-class research center found the brouhaha over O'Toole's charges discomforting. Imanishi-Kari spent a decade with her career on hold disputing the misconduct charge. O'Toole, having blown the whistle, found herself completely ostracized by the scientific community and spent a good part of the decade looking for a job. The Office of Scientific Integrity and the NIH took so long to address the charges that the scientific and medical communities require mass sedation and exposure to uninterrupted elevator music whenever the O'Toole case is mentioned.

Now that the charges of fraud have been thrown out some say the O'Toole case proves that government cannot enforce ethics in scientific research. The mere fact that it took ten years to resolve the case surely proves that is so.

The harder lesson to be learned from the tragedy of the O'Toole case is that the emphasis on government policy should not be on investigating and punishing scientific fraud but on preventing it. By the time someone is lying about his or her research results or stealing someone else's ideas, public policy and morals have already failed.

Currently the federal government requires that all those receiving federal research grants from the National Institutes of Health get training in research ethics. What the training should be, who should do it, and how it ought be evaluated are a complete mystery. More serious and systematic attention to methods for preventing unethical research is the best way to avoid the devastating human and personal costs associated with bureaucratic and legal efforts to respond once a whistle gets blown.

Misconduct

Is it impossible to say what constitutes misconduct in the practice of science? On first glance this position seems, at best, ludicrous. How could an activity such as science, conducted according to the most demanding standards of evidence and proof, be one in which misbehavior is incapable of characterization? In the absence of a definition of misconduct, the charlatans and quacks, frauds and fakes, nuts and the zealots, miscreants and butchers have as much right to lay claim to the mantle of scientific expertise as anyone else. Since anything does not go in the name of science, it must be possible to narrow down the scientific enterprise to a core set of aims, practices, and norms. Anything outside this core must be suspect as misconduct.

At worst, claims that scientific misconduct defy definition appear self-serving. Those who argue only scientists can understand what it is to do science correctly or recognize misconduct, risk placing science at the far end of an epistemological spectrum bounded by the intuitive and the mystical. An activity in which misconduct is only in the eye of the beholder, or a guild of beholders, is an activity that risks being dismissed as both overly insular and dogmatic.

Matters are not so simple, however, when the subject is defining misconduct in science. The aims, practices, and norms that constitute science are often based on textbook accounts and autobiographies. It is easy for commissions and members of congress to become confused when the basis of their claims about science are idealized reconstructions of the sort familiar from movies, textbooks, and documentaries.

The sterile, stylized version of scientific practice found in autobiographies and high school textbooks is inaccurate. The practice of science is messy. It is full of luck, emotion, ambition, odd customs, and quirks. Or, in other words, the products of science are admirable and impressive; the process by which they are made is sometimes neither. So, if it is true that science must be included along with legislation and sausages as things about which it is often better to know less than more about how they are made, where does that leave the hunt for a definition of misconduct? Oddly, it leaves the problem squarely in the lap of the scientific community.

Many, many years ago my teacher, the philosopher of science

and mathematician Ernest Nagel, remarked to me that people often expected too much of definitions. He said that while it was not always clear when a man with only a little hair ought be called bald, it was certainly true that the world was full of bald and hairy men. Bald men know who they are. So it is with scientific misconduct. Bad practitioners know who they are and so do their peers.

The place to look for definitions of misconduct in the practice of anything including science, is not to principles first and surely not to principles alone. No simple codes, values, or norms govern the practice of science. Simple moral values and maxims run aground when actual research practice turns to placebos, randomization, blinding, trade secrets, and patent issues. Anyone who tries to navigate the practice of science with a few simple values and principles will not get very far.

However, there are instances of misconduct so obvious that no one inside science disputes them. When someone paints a mouse in order to claim experimental success, does not run experiments but reports data supposedly derived from them, holds off publishing negative results until all stock and equity holdings have been sold, steals someone else's data and publishes them as their own, uses subjects incapable of giving their consent, or coerces subjects into participating in experiments, misconduct exists. Definitions of scientific misconduct do not suffer from an inability to circumvent relativism when it comes to fundamental values. They suffer from a lack of connection with the real world of science. To be useful and credible, principles must arise from an intimate knowledge of a practice rather then from efforts by outsiders to impose them on the practice.

The best hope for defining misconduct in science is to begin in the trenches not in the clouds. Principles and ideals that are not derived from actual cases will not only fail to engage the minds of those they are intended to shape, but will be difficult if not impossible to enforce. So far, those engaged in battles over scientific misconduct have been content to argue about abstractions. But there are plenty of all too real cases from which much can be learned about the difference between misconduct and the ordinary course of scientific research. Efforts to explain, prevent, and punish misconduct must merge theoretical discussion with close analyses of actual cases of right and wrong conduct. The only way the scientific community is going to focus on any definition of misconduct is if it is one that is recognizable, readily applicable, and taken seriously by those who are most knowledgeable about the practice of science.

In Industry We Should Trust?

As various Republican members of congress trip over themselves for the opportunity to disparage Bill Clinton's ethics, they are also competing to prove who hates government bureaucracy the most.

The latest charge from deconstructionists such as Rick Santorum, Orrin Hatch, and Phil Gramm is that defenders of bureaucracies like the Food and Drug Administration, the Occupational Health and Safety Administration, the Department of Agriculture are resorting to scaremongering.

Bureaucracy bashing makes for cheap political thrills in America. In the bad old days when Communism loomed, government bashers had to zip their lips. Who would do battle with the fiendish Reds if government were dismantled? Now that Marxism is just a memory it seems safe for troglodytes to lurch out from the ideological bog to tell us that the safety and health of the citizenry will be secure in the hands of the captains of industry. Not likely.

The biggest threats facing your health today are contagious diseases and unhealthy lifestyles. If you think the captains of the free market give much of a hoot about either consider two recent reports, one about AIDS and the contamination of our blood supply with the HIV virus in the early 1980s, the other an examination of the records of the Brown and Williamson Tobacco Corporation's 30-year plot to fight off tougher regulation of cigarettes.

The Institute of Medicine of the National Academy of Sciences issued a long-awaited report about how more than 8,000 hemophiliacs using blood products to prevent bleeding and 12,000 blood transfusion recipients were infected with HIV in the early 1980s. The expert panel concluded that ". . . the absence of incentives, as well as the lack of a countervailing force to advocate blood product safety, contributed to the plasma fractionation industry's slow rate of progress." In plain English, the panel found that the health care system and the blood product industry failed to move quickly to prevent the transmission of HIV to those who received blood and blood products because no regulatory agencies made them do so. Why was that? Because during the 1980s the Reagan administration was not interested in tough regulatory oversight.

The tobacco revelations are equally horrific. The July 13, 1996 issue of the *Journal of the American Medical Association* was entirely devoted to the disclosure of secret internal documents from Brown and Williamson, the third largest tobacco company in America, showing that they have known for 30 years that nicotine is addictive and that smoking causes cancer. The hypocritical drug peddlers who run the cigarette industry continue to insist that there is no reliable evidence that their product is addictive, that it kills, or that the hundreds of billions of dollars spent each year on tobacco-related illness and disability has anything to do with what they sell.

How do they get away with such patent claptrap? The tobacco lobby has prevented the FDA and other agencies from regulating tobacco as a lethal drug for decades.

Ignore the ideological mewling and political posturing over federal regulation of health and safety. Think about what the blood and tobacco industries have done for the past three decades and ask yourself in an age of AIDS, Ebola, hantavirus, virulent E. coli, and Lyme disease whether you feel safer with or without a "bureaucrat" looking over industry's shoulder?

The FDA Will Bury You!

Can the federal government's premier regulatory agency, the Food and Drug Administration, survive the collapse of the Soviet Union? What, you fail to see a connection between the former Evil Empire and the federal agency once run by a bearded, bespectacled doctor many in Congress believed to be Evil Incarnate? Well, tighten your intellectual seatbelt, pal, we're going for a ride.

Last year I spent a day in Washington, D.C. It is an especially peculiar place to visit. The streets around the Capitol teem with carefully coiffed, well-dressed, pearly toothed public servants. They are hell-bent on putting themselves out of work. Everywhere I went, from the General Accounting Office, to the FDA, to the Congressional Budget Office the bureaucrats in charge of protecting your health and safety were despondent. Why was Congress so intent upon destroying them? I tried to tell them it was the Russkies.

In the 1960s scraggly hippies descended on Washington with the intent of levitating the Pentagon and shifting power from the Beltway elite to the people. They were branded traitors, scum, and worse. A generation later the same goals minus the Pentagon levitation are espoused by a horde of young zealots, but the devotees of libertarian anarchy are hailed as heroes. Maybe the Yippies should have worn ties instead of tie-dye?

But I digress from the FDA and mother Russia. The key difference between the hostility shown the anarchist tendencies of the left in the 1960s and the enthusiasm for anarchist tendencies of the right today is the absence of an external threat to the nation. In the 1960s downsizing the government meant leaving you and me exposed to the malevolent intentions of an armed-to-the-hilt Soviet Union. The presence of the Soviet Union had a magnetic effect, it pulled us together.

I know, I know, what's all this got to do with the FDA? Well, Americans have always had a hard time agreeing on what it is that makes life worthwhile. Different cultures, religions, a broad spectrum of social, economic, and ethnic differences leave us scratching our heads at what our neighbor thinks is a pleasant way to spend a Sunday morning. The Soviet Union obscured all this. It was a humongous threat whether you believed in God, UFOs, or the NFL. A big opponent needed a big national government to take it on. And a big national government could also house an FDA and a dozen other regulatory agencies devoted to pursuing the public interest of those bound by a common threat.

Then the Soviet Union fell apart. Americans returned to their pre-cold war, pre-World War squabbling. They again see each other as having so little in common that they are content to let Congress dismantle agencies such as the FDA, whose mission is to protect them all. Without Brezhnev, Khruschev, and the rest of the dour dictators of international communism to kick around anymore there is no enthusiasm for the likes of the FDA. Hey Nikita, buddy, do us bleeding hearts some good and pound your shoe on a table and threaten to bury us just for the sake of the federal bureaucracy.

Lab Rats Put On a Few Ounces

Watching your weight? In the blubbery nation that is America where McDonald's thinks that what the middle-aged need in their lives is dead cow garnished with mustard, obesity is a major problem. What you may not have realized is that human beings are not alone in their battle against the bulge. The white rat, the most famous critter in the scientific laboratory, has, over the past several decades, become a tub too. While the bloated state of rodents may not be high on your list of things to worry about, the fact that the animals which make up the gold standard for so much medical, toxicological, and scientific research are bulging out all over is a weighty matter for your health and safety.

Richard Wassersug, a professor in the school of medicine at Dalhousie University in Nova Scotia, has taken on the role of the Richard Simmons of ratdom. Writing in *Natural History,* Wassersug notes that 50 years ago the ancestors of today's lab rats rarely weighed a pound. Today's beefy version cannot see the toenails on any of their four legs because they often weigh more than two pounds. The added mass not only makes your average rat an easy mark for pants ads that offer a bit more room where it is needed, it is not been good for rat longevity.

In 1970, 70 percent of your otherwise healthy rats hanging out in the lab lived two years. Only 10 percent of today's much porkier population persist this long.

So why all the bulk? Wassersug suggests two reasons. Today's lab rats can eat as much as they like. Our furry little friends always have a dish of chow around the old cage and no one is yet marketing "wide-load" magnets to discourage them from sticking their whiskers in whenever they wish.

The other reason is more subtle. Breeders make more money if they can produce a rat that is on the larger end of the spectrum since, in many studies, it is easier to work with a bigger animal. So the companies that supply lab animals have been choosing a bigger, fatter, rat.

All right you say, so lab rats are getting fatter. Maybe someone needs to devise miniature Thighmasters or Abdominizers for them. Let ad geniuses come up with an infomercial that will convince these lardballs to get off their tails and sweat. But, otherwise, who really cares if gluttonous lab rats die young?

Hey, show some sympathy to a fellow life form struggling to keep those buns hard, will you? It so happens that a fat rat not only dies earlier but is more prone to developing tumors and other health problems. If a company or a scientist is trying to figure out whether something is safe for you to eat or a medicine might have dangerous side effects, a lab rat that is far more likely than it once was to spontaneously get sick and grow frail is a lab rat that is not able to function as well as a sentinel to protect your health. The more likely it is for rats to get sick, the harder it is to find the cause.

But lest you leave this space fearful that a fat rat may not be the best predictor of what your toilet cleanser or hair conditioner may actually be doing to your well-being, I espy good news among the folds of rat fat. Perhaps the rotund rat of today is still a good model to use to see what the side effects might be of daily diet of beef jerky, coffee, and Cheez Whiz. For we, like the rats, are heavier than our grandparents. As a result our fat little furry friends may be a better reflection of the risks and dangers of what we ingest than we would care to admit when looking in a mirror.

Research in an Emergency

No matter where you turn in America, race matters. Want to know what is going on in the corporate offices at Texaco, in courtroom trials of or about celebrities in California, Pennsylvania, and New York, in the streets of St. Petersburg, Florida, in battles all over this nation about housing, school vouchers, immigration, and zoning? Start with race.

You might think the one place where race might not matter is on a stretcher in the emergency room or in the back of a speeding ambulance. Think again. The decision by the Food and Drug Administration to permit some forms of research in emergency circumstances without informed consent shows how much race matters, even when the subject is saving lives.

For years those working in emergency rooms, as well as those who make drugs and medical devices intended for use in these places, have complained about the difficulties of finding new and better treatments for those who suddenly and unexpectedly find themselves dying, disabled, or incapacitated. If you were to be the victim of massive head trauma as a result of a fall or automobile accident, burst a blood vessel deep in your brain, accidentally swallow a poisonous mushroom, be infected with a rare strain of "flesh eating" bacteria, overdose on PCP, homemade liquor, or tainted heroin, or suffer a sudden unexpected bout of severe asthma, you could very well end up dead. Medicine has treatments to offer for each of these emergencies but, regrettably, they often do not work well and sometimes do not work at all. The only way to change that is to conduct research in these emergency settings. Until recently if you could not consent, such research was against the law.

Now, the FDA has approved rules that say that in life-threatening situations where there are either no available proven treatments or the existing treatments are "unsatisfactory," where research on animals shows that a new drug, device, or treatment holds some hope of benefit, and where it is impossible to get consent from a family member or surrogate, then research may be done on a person without their permission. The FDA insists that any such experiment be cleared by a local committee at the clinic, hospital, or medical center where research without consent will be done. Communities are supposed to be notified about what is going to be done before any research without consent is started, but it is not at all clear, short of sky-writing, sound trucks, or the construction of downtown Jumbotrons, exactly what the FDA has in mind.

Which brings us to race. The FDA rules have created a huge stir in minority communities all over this nation. In the city where I live, Philadelphia, many African Americans and Hispanics are expressing their fears about what will happen if doctors can legally experiment upon people without their consent. Why?

The answer quite simply is race. Race has always played a huge role in American medicine. Many Americans can still remember a time when hospitals were segregated both by patient and physician. Race is still one of the first things mentioned in presenting a case at hospital rounds or in taking a family history. And most African Americans know that race has played a key role in the history of medical experimentation in this country since it is the reason why so many black people have been forced, tricked, or duped into immoral experiments, most especially the notorious Tuskegee study in which rural black men were left untreated for syphilis starting in 1932 and up to 1971 even when a cure, penicillin, became available in the late 1940s. Research on blacks in prisons, poor neighborhoods, and on the Bowery was so extensive in the 1960s and early 1970s that some black children were warned not to go near large medical centers at night for fear that doctors would snatch them for experiments.

It makes good sense to let some forms of research proceed in emergencies without the consent of subjects. But, it makes no sense to pretend that race does not matter in determining how such a policy will be received. The only way to make sure that minorities do not come to further distrust a health care system that has exploited or betrayed them in the past is to make sure that the committees charged with approving research without consent have many minority voices.

The Return of Thalidomide

Thalidomide. The word practically jumped right off the page of the informed consent form for a proposed study at the University of Pennsylvania. Researchers at Penn and other medical schools are eager to see whether thalidomide might help in the treatment of patients dying of AIDS. The drug might help combat the painful mouth ulcers that make it impossible for those with AIDS to eat, leading to malnutrition and wasting. What caught my eye was that the researchers were seeking permission to test one of the most notorious and controversial drugs in the history of modern medicine. They wanted to try the drug in both men and women. Thalidomide is one of the most dangerous drugs that could possibly be given to a woman.

Thalidomide was first brought on the market in Europe in the 1950s as a sleeping pill. By the early 1960s it was being prescribed to women in Sweden, Germany, Britain, France, Australia, and Japan to relieve the nausea associated with pregnancy. Then, disaster struck. Nearly 12,000 babies were born throughout the world with severe birth defects. Many were born with no arms. Others with ghastly malformations of their heads and bodies. Thalidomide was to blame. It is one of the most powerful causes of birth defects known to medical science. By allowing the drug to go on the market for pregnant women without adequate animal and human testing, thousands of kids were born dead, retarded, or with severe physical deformities.

As I looked through the informed consent form it became clear that the researchers involved in the study knew all this. Still, the danger the drug poses to a developing fetus did not stop them from wanting to test it in women.

Federal law requires researchers to allow fair access to both men and women in research trials. Since both men and women get AIDS and since both sexes die from the wasting and malnutrition caused by the disease, both sexes, the researchers reasoned, ought to be included in the study.

The very drug that led to the exclusion of so many women from so many scientific studies for so many years is now back as something women should have a right to try. After the thalidomide disaster, the

FDA, other regulatory agencies, and those designing experiments did everything they could to keep women who had any chance of becoming pregnant out of research studies of new drugs. It was not until pressure mounted from women outraged about the lack of female subjects in medical research studies that something was done.

Women should have the same right to be involved in experiments as men. However, equal opportunity needs to be limited when there is a danger of causing tremendous harm.

When experimental drugs are known to be dangerous to an embryo or fetus, the first group of subjects studied ought to be men along with women who cannot become pregnant. Before exposing large numbers of fertile women to a drug known to be incredibly toxic to fetuses, it makes sense to see if it can do any good in people who cannot become pregnant. Everyone deserves a fair shot at the benefits of medical research. The exception must be that if a drug is known to cause birth defects and fetal deaths, then even though it means women will not have the same initial chance to try a new drug as men, those who cannot become pregnant should go first.

Acne, Accutane, and Ethics

When the health interests of mothers and babies collide, whose interests should win? A study in the *New England Journal of Medicine* shows that with the right combination of government regulation and responsible corporate conduct, both can come out ahead.

In 1982, Accutane, a synthetic vitamin derivative, became available in the United States for the treatment of severe, disfiguring acne. It quickly became apparent that while the drug was effective, it is extremely dangerous to a developing fetus. Almost 30 percent of babies born to women who used Accutane during pregnancy had moderate or severe birth defects of their bones, heart, brain, or spinal cord. By 1987 there were 78 confirmed cases where Accutane was known to be the cause of a malformed or stillborn infant.

The high rate of birth defects led the FDA to act. In 1988 after reviewing the evidence from dermatologists, pediatricians, and patients, the agency decided to allow Accutane to stay on the market. But the FDA insisted that the manufacturer, Hoffman-La Roche, agree to commit itself to an intensive program to educate doctors and women of child-bearing age about the need to prevent pregnancy while taking Accutane.

The company agreed. A sincere effort was made to warn women about the risk of birth defects. A first-rate educational program was designed and distributed to every American doctor who prescribed Accutane. Information on the importance of pregnancy tests for prospective users, contraception use, menstruation and fertility, bluntly worded patient inserts, and regular updates for doctors and pharmacists was widely distributed.

The Pregnancy Prevention Program worked. A study by Dr. Alan A. Mitchell and colleagues at Boston University's School of Public Health showed that women using the drug understand the risk of birth defects and the need to avoid pregnancy. The number of women who got the message "was virtually universal" the study finds. And the message led to behavioral change. While the average rate of pregnancy among women age 15 to 44 is 109 per thousand, the rate among Accutane users is 8.8. Only one half of one percent of the 148,000 women surveyed who were sexually active failed to use contraception or some means of birth control.

These numbers are incredible. Anyone working in the fields of sexuality, birth control, venereal disease, or HIV education knows how hard it is to get people to change their behavior, even for a short period of time, when the behavior involves sex. The survey shows that when government and the private sector are on the same page the public can come out a winner.

But the survey of Accutane users also showed that a real commitment of energy, money, and resources is needed to achieve informed consent. This is a lesson our nation would do well to heed as we think about whether or not we really want to heed the call of some bureaucracy bashers who wish to dismantle the FDA. Policy makers also need to keep this success story in mind in thinking about what it really costs to put a new drug on the market that fertile women might take. It will be a tragedy if the next generation of drugs beneficial for women but dangerous to fetuses pit mothers against their children because there is no watchdog agency or funds available to do what is needed to protect them both.

Give 'Em an Inch

Raymond Hintz, a pediatric endocrinologist at Stanford University Medical Center, has very mixed feelings about his research. In a way he hoped the experiment he was conducting would fail. But it didn't. Hintz has found a way to make some young kids grow taller. He has also created a large moral problem as a result.

Hintz says that by using synthetic growth hormone he can add two to three inches of height to very short children. We now must face the question of whether medicine should be in the business of making short people taller.

Hintz and his associates gave synthetic growth hormone by daily injection to 51 kids over a number of years. Children enrolled in the study produced normal amounts of growth hormone, but nevertheless lagged at least two years behind other kids their age in terms of height. At the rate they were growing this group of children, while not dwarves, would wind up in the shortest 2 percent of the population.

Kids who got the genetically engineered hormone grew more than similar children who did not get shots. About half the kids who got hormone grew an additional two inches. A few gained four or five inches beyond what their growth curves would have predicted. However, a quarter of the kids who had been through hundreds of injections got absolutely no benefit.

Still, Hintz's work shows that for some short kids, a boost of artificial growth hormone might add a couple more inches to their height. While Hintz's work is only a single study, you can be sure there are plenty of parents and kids out there who will want growth hormone shots. Should pediatricians honor their requests?

There are roughly 20,000 to 30,000 kids who in any given year fall far below average in terms of growth. That is a lot of customers. The market for supplying this group with artificial growth hormone is estimated at around $400 million per year. Aggressive marketing could make tens of thousands of other kids uneasy about their height. A few years ago, the vice president for sales and marketing of the company that makes the best-selling version of synthetic growth hormone was indicted in a kickback scheme to get doctors to refer patients for growth hormone treatments. It would not take an advertising genius to devise a campaign that could get a lot of kids and parents frantic about getting shots.

There are those who will say that if kids or their parents want to take growth hormone and doctors are willing to prescribe it, it is nobody else's business. But the ethical problem is that preying on the fears and stigma associated with shortness could easily become a business that gets out of hand. The pediatric community needs to do some quick thinking about the degree to which it will promote growth hormone for short children, and the extent to which it is committed to try and convince parents and kids that there is nothing wrong with being shorter than average. Without some clear, enforceable guidelines, the potential for abuse of growth hormone injections in children is very, very large.

Betrayal of Trust

There would seem to be little doubt that individuals institution-alized with severe mental impairment due to illness or injury must be counted among the ranks of the potentially most vulnerable of those who might be involved in biomedical research. Yet, those who have severe Alzheimer's disease, schizophrenia, autism, depression, and other forms of mental illness that leave them impaired and dependent upon others do not have the same level of protection as do other groups involved in biomedical research. Special federal regulations govern the participation of such vulnerable groups as children, fe-tuses, and prisoners in biomedical research. However, there are no special federal regulations governing the involvement of those with severe mental illness in research. Should special rules exist? And even if they were written, are they likely to afford adequate protection of the human rights, welfare, and dignity of the mentally impaired who act as research subjects?

Many people believe that it was the discovery of the cruel and barbarous experiments conducted by German scientists and doctors in the concentration camps during World War II that led to the de-mand for the creation of ethical standards governing human re-search. But that is not so. And, some of the American scientists who were involved in the radiation experiments on human subjects spon-sored by various federal agencies during the late 1940s and 1950s maintain that the ethical standards which existed in those days were entirely different from those that exist today. But that is not so ei-ther.

In actuality, the cruel and lethal experiments on those in the concentration camps of Poland, France, and Germany were held to be in obvious violation of the prevailing standards of research ethics by the Nuremberg tribunal and various national and international medical organizations. The German defendants invoked national se-curity, the special circumstances of war, and the fact that there sub-jects were doomed to die as reasons why they did not get the informed consent and voluntary participation of their subjects. The American experts called upon to testify at Nuremberg rejected these excuses. Dr. Andrew Ivy testified that voluntary participation and informed consent were central to the ethical conduct of research and could never be waived or ignored. The Nuremberg tribunal agreed.

The Nuremberg Code, which was actually part of the decision of the military tribunal examining Nazi war crimes, was published in 1949. The Code did not articulate a new level of ethical protection for those involved in medical research so much as it did reaffirm an old one. The key protections outlined in the Code and in the subsequent Declaration of Helsinki of the World Medical Association concerning the ethics of research, which was ratified in 1964, reaffirmed that informed consent and voluntary participation of subjects were essential to all ethical biomedical research. They also held that researchers should not conduct research in which they knew that subjects were certain or very likely to be disabled, injured, or killed.

Those, such as some of those who conducted radiation experiments involving the death of prisoners in Washington and Oregon in the 1950s, who argue that the ethical standards that prevail now did not exist then, are simply wrong. The Nuremberg Code and the proceedings of the Nuremberg trials make it clear that informed consent was just as much a part of the ethics of biomedical research in 1944 as it is in 1998.

Unfortunately, the Nuremberg Code and the declarations of ethical codes by various international medical organizations did not have much of an impact in the United States. Indeed, as the distinguished Harvard anesthesiologist Henry Beecher would find to his dismay in his landmark paper, "Ethics and Clinical Research," published in the *New England Journal of Medicine* in 1966, and as former Secretary of Energy Hazel O' Leary would learn in 1994, there was a great deal of research conducted in the late 1940s, 1950s, and 1960s that did not live up to the ideals and moral requirements expressed in the various codes of ethics and international conventions issued during these same years.

The recognition of the need for more oversight and regulation for those participating in biomedical research only arose in the early late 1970s. The revelation in 1973 of the Tuskegee study led to a public outcry concerning the ethics of human experimentation.

The Tuskegee study, which began in 1932, was a 40-year experiment to learn about the clinical course of syphilis by studying poor, ill-educated African American males in Alabama who were left untreated and uninformed about the nature of their disease. The study was funded by the U.S. Public Health Service and depended upon the active participation of government, state and county doctors, public officials, and nurses. Even after penicillin was widely available, the subjects in this study were not given the drug but were deliberately deceived and given placebo treatments so that more data could be collected.

It was congressional anger over the discovery that the Tuskegee study had gone on for so many years with federal support that led to the creation of a special commission, the National Commission for the Protection of Human Subjects of Biomedical And Behavioral Research, which issued its findings, commonly referred to as the Belmont Report, in 1978. This report recommended specific rules be put in place for research involving human subjects using federal funds. It also called for the creation of special committees, now called institutional review boards or IRBs, to review the risks and benefits of research proposals before participation was offered to potential subjects. And the report outlined special rules for protecting the interests of those it termed vulnerable populations among whom were included children, fetuses, and the institutionalized mentally infirm.

Many of these recommendations were enacted into federal law in 1981. CFR 45.46 calls for the creation of IRBs to review each research protocol using human subjects for which federal financial support is being sought. The law also requires IRBs to review the informed consent forms used with research protocols, to insure that subject selection in research is fair and equitable and to monitor compliance by researchers in gaining informed consent from their subjects. Special regulations were written for experimentation on fetuses and children.

Thus, today there are really two sorts of protections afforded those involved in human research. Informed consent is to be obtained from every potential subject. Those being approached about participating in a study are to receive all the information they wish about the study, a discussion of the all options available to them for treatment, and to understand that they can decline to participate or withdraw as a participant at any time without penalty.

Each research project is to be reviewed by an IRB among whose members is to be at least one person not formally affiliated with the institution where the research is to be done. Those subjects who are drawn from so-called vulnerable groups may be involved in research only when the research has as its goal some therapeutic benefit for the subject, when the risks involved are minimal, and when a surrogate has given consent for their participation in the case of minor children.

There are no special restrictions about the kind of research that can be conducted with subjects who are mentally ill. While surrogate or substitute consent must be obtained for those deemed incompetent, the risk-benefit ratio and goals of research are the same for those who are mentally ill as they would be for any other person.

Treating the mentally ill, even the institutionalized mentally ill the same as any other group in terms of the kind of research that they can be involved in, may allow the mentally ill to benefit from access to better drugs or medical devices. It means that researchers face less red tape and paperwork in trying to conduct research on mental illness. It may even minimize the stigma associated with mental illness by not singling out the mentally ill for special treatment under federal regulations. But it also means that to the extent some of those with mental illness are especially vulnerable due to organic dysfunction or institutionalization there are no special provisions in place to insure their rights and well-being.

This situation should be changed. Not the least because of recent instances of exploitation and mistreatment of those with mental illness recruited into research.

Subjects with severe mental illness have been allowed to decompensate in order to assess the therapeutic value of new treatments, required to "wash out" (go off their medications) as a precondition for participation in studies, or subjected, in the case of elderly persons with severe dementia, to round after round of new drugs with powerful side effects in the hope of finding a cure. Addicts have been lied to in the case of persons from Southeast Asia who were given various experimental interventions in the hope of finding a remedy for their drug abuse without true informed consent. The Congress, the FDA, the National Institutes of Health, and the federal government should reopen the issue of whether special regulations are in order.

The twin protections of informed consent and IRB review are not always adequate for protecting the dignity and well-being of subjects who are not mentally ill when they become involved in experimental research. Time after time stories hit the front page of researchers conducting tests of new therapies such as the Jarvik 7 artificial heart, pig liver transplants, extra corporeal membrane oxygenation on young children, bone marrow transplants on kids with congenital disorders, and lung transplants using lobes of lung removed from living donors where IRBs seem to have done little except rubber stamp dubious protocols and the informed consent of the subjects is, in actuality, the product of nothing more than desperation on the part of subjects and their families.

It is not clear that informed consent and review by IRBs are sufficient protections for those involved in human research. If so they are plainly not enough for high-risk research involving persons with moderate or severe mental illness. Research involving decompensation or "washing out" should be reviewed by national rather than local IRBs. Any study that involves institutionally mentally infirm subjects should be subject to audit and random site visits by national authorities. Parents, patients, and relatives of those with mental illness must be adequately represented on review committees or funding agency review boards so that the interests and welfare of those with mental illness are adequately reflected in the funding and review process.

It is scandal that is the source of the current system for protecting the rights of those involved in biomedical research. But scandals are an unacceptable stimulus for further thinking about how best to advance research on mental illness in a manner consistent with the interests, welfare, and dignity of subjects. It is long since past time for issuing new rules clarifying what can and cannot be done by researchers who wish to study the mentally ill and impaired.

What We Do for Animals We Should Do for People

America has not always done what it should to insure the welfare and dignity of those who altruistically make themselves available as subjects so that medicine can learn and advance in the battle against disease and disability. As the troubling revelations of the exploitation of subjects—including children with mental retardation, the elderly, and soldiers in the 1950s and 1960s in research involving the study of radioactive substances, and the outright deception and fraud perpetrated by our government upon poor African-American men infected with syphilis in rural Alabama for four decades in the notorious Tuskegee study, this nation's ethics have not always been what they ought to have been in the area of biomedical research.

As a result of these and other scandals coming to light, a debate ensued in this nation concerning the ethics of human experimentation. We have as a society made a commitment to do better by those involved in research as subjects. And we have. But we have not done enough. It is time to revisit the adequacy of human-subject regulations in the United States for three reasons: a rapidly changing research environment that casts doubt on the adequacy of informed consent and institutional review board (IRB) review; a lack of basic information about who is involved in research; and inadequate attention to the needs of those who are most vulnerable in research contexts.

Shifts in Financing, Organization, and Purposes of Human Research

For thirty years research in the United States has been subject to policies and regulations imposed by the federal government. In the wake of scandals in the late 1960s and early 1970s, such as the Tuskegee syphilis study, the Brooklyn Chronic Disease Hospital cancer study, and the Willowbrook hepatitis vaccine trials, two types of protection were created for those recruited to serve as subjects in biomedical research. The first, informed consent, requires that participation in research be voluntary, informed, and freely chosen. The second, review by local IRBs, insures that the scientific merit, risk/benefit ratio, and informed consent documents associated with individual research proposals are approved by the peers of those seeking permission to undertake research. Local review of recruitment and consent practices, with relatively little centralized oversight by federal agencies, was held to be most consistent with American values, easier to implement, and most responsive to the style of federally sponsored, project- and research-oriented funding that characterized biomedical inquiry in this country in the 1970s and early 1980s.

The twin protections of informed consent and IRB review have served subjects well. Some of the most egregious scandals in our own history of research involving human subjects, such as the racism, deception and callous indifference to human life of the Tuskegee study, could not take place under the current system of regulations. However, the existing system of regulations has not been seriously revised or revisited since 1981. In the more than a decade-and-a-half since the rules were last revised a number of changes have occurred in the conduct, organization, and financing of human research.

Privatization

One of the most startling changes has been the shift from public to private sources in the funding of human-subject research. Private industry is now the major source of funding for biomedical research in the United States. Since 1980, industry's share of U.S. biomedical research and development rose from 31 percent to 46 percent, while NIH's share dropped from 40 percent to 32 percent. The dramatic increase of industry funding of biotechnology and clinical research is reflected in university research budgets as well. Industry support of all university research has nearly doubled in the last decade, from 4 percent to 7 percent. More than a third of the authors in a recent sample of leading biomedical journals had at least one potential conflict of interest as a result of receiving private support or holding a financial interest in the drug or device being studied. Privatization of support for biomedical research has led to some obvious problems and challenges.

Access to information for subjects, researchers and the public is emerging as a problem. Commercial motives are fueling the content and direction of an increasing number of biomedical research projects, resulting in more secrecy in research protocols. As the battle between the University of California, San Francisco, and the Knoll Pharmaceutical Company (formerly Boots Co.) over the right to publish findings that did not reflect positively on a new drug proves, private concerns can and do exercise control over what researchers can publish.

When a UCSF researcher found that Synthroid, a widely used drug, which costs Americans $600 million per year, was biologically equivalent to the much less-expensive generics, the company suppressed publication of the findings and threatened UCSF with a lawsuit to keep the study from being published. It was only when the company decided to yield early in 1997, almost two years later, to the mounting outcry from the medical community, that the data appeared. Not publishing legitimate findings is a betrayal of the obligation owed to those who participate in human research.

The privatization of research has led to another shift in human-subject research. Private concerns frequently seek subjects in order to test new drugs or devices they wish to bring to the marketplace. Federally funded research is far less likely to be driven by commercial considerations than privately sponsored research. This means that human subjects may be asked to carry risks or face the burdens of participation in a research trial when not fully understanding that the research is being undertaken with a commercial purpose in mind.

I have seen many protocols come before IRBs on which I have served over the past few years where the drug in question was being tested so that a particular pharmaceutical firm could enter into a lucrative market where many other similar or nearly identical drugs already existed. Subjects may not always be informed of the fact that the researcher requesting their participation in a study stands to gain financially from their consent. Nor do they always understand why a study is being done or what will be done with the results of a study sponsored by a private concern.

The shift toward more private than public support of research raises questions about the adequacy of local IRB review, which plays such a key role in the federal oversight of human research. IRBs may not always know what the conflicts of interest are that exist due to ties between researchers and private funding sources. They may themselves, be in a conflicted position, trying to do the right thing by the subjects but feeling tremendous pressure not to alienate those who provide the bulk of support for a particular center or department within an institution. Indeed, some forms of research, when conducted entirely with private support, may not fall under the legal aegis of IRB review.

The privatization of research has been accompanied by another major change in the nature of biomedical research. The era of the single investigator conducting work with a set of subjects at one institution is coming to an end.

Multiple Investigators at Multiple Locations Imperil Informed Consent and Strain IRBs

Today, many subjects in research participate in "multi-site" studies. These are studies that involve many investigators recruiting subjects at many different institutions and locations, often across national boundaries. Multi-site research was not the model that shaped the creation of local IRBs, the linchpin of peer review for approving human research. And it is becoming increasingly obvious that local IRBs cannot handle some of the issues that arise in publicly and privately funded multi-site research. One such example is the large-scale misconduct that, when discovered in 1994, cast suspicion over the integrity of the National Surgical Adjuvant Breast and Bowel Project (NSABP), the single most important source of information that women facing surgery for breast cancer have available for themselves and their doctors.

Dr. Roger Poisson of St. Luc hospital in Montreal fraudulently enrolled at least 100 subjects into this study. His patients constituted 16 percent of the study population. Researchers in this multi-center study were paid on the basis of the number of patients enrolled. Successful recruiters such as Poisson were also given authorship on key papers from the NSABP.

No aspect of the fraud that occurred in this study was detected and reported by any IRB, even though there were tremendous variations in the informed consent forms used by participating institutions to recruit subjects. And no IRB member was ever asked to audit or debrief any subject or investigator in the study at any point during the many years it ran or even after the fraud in Montreal was discovered.

Multi-site research poses real challenges for the current system. Local IRBs may or may not be coordinating their review of informed consent documents. Investigators conducting the same study at different places must often contend with inconsistent demands and requests by IRBs. And subjects may or may not receive a core or minimal set of information about a study for which they are being recruited, depending on the zealousness and competency of the IRB. Indeed, some research is conducted under the auspices of IRBs that are hired for the sole purpose of reviewing studies, which raises questions about their ability to assess and monitor local conditions and the needs of particular subjects for information or special protections in particular places.

A Lack of Basic Information

IRBs lack the manpower, budget, or time to do much more than review written research protocols and check informed consent forms. In my experience I have never met an IRB member who has spent any serious amount of time debriefing subjects. No IRBs I know of spend any time visiting with researchers to track the implementation of informed consent or to assess the nature of the ethical problems that have actually arisen in the course of conducting research.

IRBs are trapped by paperwork. They almost never have the time or the mission to talk with subjects. Thus, they remain uninformed about the extent to which what they require on paper in the way of informed consent is actually put into practice or valued by the subjects of that research.

There is no systematic collection of data for the demographics of participants in human research, which compounds the burden that IRBs face. We mandate far more stringent data collection and monitoring regarding animal subjects than we do human subjects.

No one can say what the workload is that IRBs face, what the demographics are of those asked to participate in research, or what the actual demographic content is of those volunteering to be in research in any given month or year because no data about any of these matters is systematically collected or published. If there are trends involving the participation of women, poor people, the mentally ill, or Native Americans, or any other group, no one knows because no historical data exists about demographics or the nature of those involved in human research. We have more information about the fate of animals in research than people and that simply should not be.

Nor is there any systematic debriefing done of those who have participated in research or who have acted as surrogates for those not competent to consent for themselves. This means that IRBs must operate in a vacuum when issues of discrimination, fair access, or bias arise with respect to research protocols. It also means that there is no way to check whether IRBs actually do emphasize in their work the kinds of issues that are most important to those who actually serve as human subjects.

Nor is there any systematically collected data on IRB performance. Audits of IRBs are rare and are usually triggered by the hint or allegation of a problem. The ability of IRB members to monitor the actual conduct of research, and their skill in doing so, is not demonstrable by existing means of oversight of the IRB system. Many subjects remain unaware of what to do if they feel that they have been mistreated or wronged in the course of research. And by having the major federal office responsible for the protection of research subjects, the OPRR, located at the NIH, it may not be possible for that agency to have the kind of independence and autonomy necessary to monitor both private and publicly-sponsored research activities.

The Failure to Grapple with the Needs of Vulnerable Populations in Human Research

For many years it has been well understood that not all subjects in human research can look out for their own interests. When people are, for various reasons, incapable of fully exercising their power of self-determination or of acting as an autonomous agent, they are at increased risk when serving as a subject because one of the two forms of protection deemed crucial for ethical experimentation, informed consent, is not available to them. Classic examples of such vulnerable subjects are children and fetuses. Special regulations govern their participation in research as they are unable to consent to participate for themselves.

In the 1990s a series of problems and scandals has arisen within some populations of research participants. These include the severely mentally ill, members of our armed forces, the senile elderly, the terminally ill, poor women, students, and those who suddenly and unexpectedly become acutely ill. There is also the very important issue of the extent to which guidelines concerning informed consent will be followed when research done by Americans or sponsored by American companies or government agencies is conducted outside our borders. Many of the subjects in studies in poor nations lack the education and even the cultural familiarity with concepts like autonomy and individual rights that would allow them to make full use of informed consent.

Experiments have been conducted on persons with mental illnesses where informed consent has been poor and the monitoring of subjects involved in studies inadequate. Complaints by a number of persons afflicted with schizophrenia and their families about studies carried out at UCLA raise some very tough questions about the adequacy of existing rules for protecting those who are made vulnerable by mental illness. Issues have arisen concerning the rights and duties that those serving the nation in active military service have in times of war and peace with respect to participation in biomedical research undertaken for military purposes. Some of those who served in the Persian Gulf conflict were exposed to vaccines and drugs under circumstances that closely resemble research without informed consent.

Patients with dementia due to Alzheimer's Disease have been routinely recruited as subjects in studies sponsored by private funds where their informed consent and handling as subjects is highly suspect, as was revealed in 1996 at the Medical College of Georgia. In these studies, study coordinators stressed payment for participation over risks and benefits, and medical supervision of subjects was scandalously inadequate. Poor women at the Medical College of South Carolina in Charleston have been duped and coerced into participating in studies aimed at decreasing drug abuse during pregnancy. Retarded children in institutions in New York have been used as subjects for research not intended to benefit or help them, leading a judge to impose a ban on all research involving institutionalized mentally retarded children in the state.

Terminally ill persons have been subject to all manner of innovative efforts of clinical therapy without adequate IRB review. One of many such examples is the use of the rapidly evolving surgical procedure for treating heart failure, sometimes known as the Batista procedure. In this procedure tissue is removed from the heart in order to increase the pumping ability of the organ. No good data exists about the safety or efficacy of the procedure. Yet it is spreading rapidly through American hospitals and surgical clinics. In part this is because under our existing regulations there is no clear-cut requirement that new and innovative surgical procedures be subject to a level of review on a par with the review mandated when a human subject is involved in the testing of a new drug or medical device.

None of these problems has been detected or reported by IRBs. Vulnerable populations are not getting the level of protection they need to ensure their informed participation in research.

Those who cannot consent, or who can do so only in a limited sense, still deserve the opportunity to participate in biomedical research. There are often benefits to be gained from participation in research, both directly for the subject and indirectly in terms of knowledge gained that can benefit others with similar conditions and debilities.

Vulnerability is not in itself a sufficient reason to deny participation in research to any person. But, there is sufficient evidence available to conclude that some groups, such as the mentally ill, the institutionalized demented elderly, and those in military service, require more protection than they are currently being afforded by existing regulations; while others, such as children, the terminally ill, and the unexpectedly acutely ill, may need more protection than they are currently being afforded by a system of local IRB review.

What Should Be Done?

There are many areas where Congress and the White House must call for greater action on the part of federal agencies and offices responsible for protecting the rights and welfare of human subjects in biomedical research. The following seven recommendations are especially important if human subjects are to get the protection they deserve.

1. Special provisions and oversight for those with cognitive and emotional impairment sufficient to interfere with their capacity for informed consent should be added to existing regulations governing human-subject research.
2. A clearer definition of research should be incorporated into existing federal regulations to insure that what is truly and obviously new, innovative, and pioneering is subject to consent and IRB review.
3. Steps should be taken to decrease the paperwork burden faced by researchers and IRBs, and to permit IRBs more time to conduct monitoring activities on research and to debrief subjects. This could be accomplished by moving the current review system in

the direction of random audits similar to those used by the IRS, FDA, and many commercial enterprises to insure quality control.

4. Standardized data on human subject participation in research as well as IRB activity should be mandated, collected, and made widely available.

5. All sources of conflicts of interest must be disclosed to IRBs, and all information necessary for the protection of human subjects must be placed in their hands regardless of commercial concerns.

6. For some categories and kinds of research involving vulnerable populations or high-risk inquiry, consideration ought be given to the creation of regional or national IRB-like review mechanisms to be added to local IRB review.

7. More audit and monitoring responsibilities should be given both to local IRBs to assess compliance with informed consent and to the OPRR at the NIH to monitor IRB performance.

Participation in medical research always carries some risk. Those who bear that risk, especially those who, for one reason or another, cannot make a decision to participate as a subject, deserve every protection society can afford them as they face those risks.

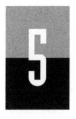

New Treatment/
New Challenges

- Should a Fetus Be a Parent?
- Tiny Mermaids
- No Deposit, No Return
- Cyber Medicine
- Rethinking the Cost of War
- Baboons and Bone Marrow
- Hearts and Minds
- Seeing Straight on Patents
- Why Say No to Life?
- Breast Cancer and BMT
- Laser Blinding

Should a Fetus Be a Parent?

In early January of 1995 a scientist in Scotland, Roger Gosden of the University of Edinburgh, announced to the media that he thought it possible to use eggs obtained from aborted fetuses to help infertile women have babies. He said he could do this by harvesting fetal ovaries and grafting them into the ovaries of infertile women. If so, the transplant would be of benefit to women who cannot make their own eggs either because they have reached menopause or because of some disorder or disease that makes their eggs abnormal. Gosden said that he had successfully transplanted fetal ovaries in mice and that he will soon be ready to try the technique using human fetal eggs.

It is nothing short of remarkable that a scientist chose to use the lay press to announce findings concerning the harvesting of fetal ovaries. But this was not the first time that researchers have circumvented the usual channels of peer review with respect to transplants aimed at helping those with incurable diseases. Announcements about the use of adrenal glands and later fetal brain tissue to try and help those with parkinsonism first came to public attention in media reports. Although some scientists complain that it is the media that stirs the pot of controversy concerning scientific advances, it is oftentimes true, especially in areas pertaining to reproduction, genetic engineering, or the use of fetal tissue, that it is scientists who seek attention, public acclaim, or a demonstration of priority before their work has undergone peer review in the professional literature.

Gosden's announcement was met with a storm of controversy. Some commentators in the United Kingdom immediately pronounced the idea of using eggs from aborted fetuses ethically repugnant. A group of British legislators said they would quickly draft a law to outlaw such transplants. The British Medical Association said it would move rapidly to create a commission to examine the issue. The tone of their announcement made it clear that they were not enthusiastic about Dr. Gosden's transplant plans.

Some American ethicists such as myself, George Annas, Mark Siegler, and many others were quick to condemn the idea as morally suspect. Two members of the medical ethics program at the University of Wisconsin, Alta Charo and Dan Wikler, were apparently so unnerved by the rapid negative reaction to Gosden's claims that they issued a call for a self-imposed moratorium on the proffering of timely opinions about fetal egg harvesting or any advance in reproductive technology.

Some did not find the idea of harvesting eggs from aborted fetuses so obviously repugnant. Nor did they believe, as Charo and Wikler argued, that they ought to muzzle their enthusiasm until a suitable period of deliberative thought had passed.

Professor John Fletcher, a distinguished theologian at the University of Virginia's Program in Biomedical Ethics, acknowledged that taking eggs from aborted fetuses might seem initially bizarre. Fletcher maintained, however, that it could help women who cannot now find willing donors to obtain eggs. Moreover, harvesting eggs from fetuses would reduce the number of women who now undergo possibly risky hormonal treatments in order to serve as egg donors. The benefits of fetal transplants might well outweigh our squeamishness about the source.

Some infertility specialists in the United States declared that those who find the idea of mining fetal eggs revolting simply fail to understand the desperation and the anguish of women who desperately want to have a child. The musings of professional worrywarts about the ethics of taking eggs from aborted fetuses pale, these doctors said, in the light of the good that can come from finding a way to allow infertile women to have babies.

The consensus of initial opinion regarding the use of fetal ovaries obtained from aborted fetuses as sources of eggs for the infertile seemed to be negative. This was different from the reaction to proposals only six years earlier to use fetal tissue from aborted fetuses for transplant research. Only right-to-life groups opposed the use of fetal tissue for transplant research, but a wide spectrum of individuals evinced concern about the use of fetal eggs and ovaries. Why the difference in stance? Are there any real moral differences between using fetal islet cells obtained from the remains of an aborted fetus to try and control insulin production in a diabetic and inserting fetal ovaries or eggs taken from the same aborted fetus in a women whose own ovaries do not function?

I think there are some important differences between the moral issues raised by the use of somatic fetal tissues and fetal germ cells. Transplanting an islet cell is not the same as transplanting an egg. One procedure might save a life. The other will create a new one. And therein lies a significant moral difference. But before looking at the ethical issue it is important to ask whether fetal ovary transplants could really be done.

All of the eggs that a woman will ever have are present by the tenth or eleventh week of fetal development. So the eggs would appear to be there for harvesting if ovaries can actually be transplanted.

A mouse is not a human being, however. Human reproduction is notoriously difficult to regulate and control. In fact, if it were not so hard, there would not be so many frustrated childless couples who cannot be helped by current medical techniques. Very little is known about the development of eggs in fetuses or about the environment necessary to allow fetal eggs to be fertilized and develop into babies. Moreover, despite some optimistic assertions to the effect that fetal ovaries may be less vulnerable to rejection by the recipient's natural immunological defense system, a woman who gets a fetal ovary might reject it unless she takes the same battery of immunosuppressive drugs that all organ transplant recipients must now endure. The few papers published on the transplantation of adult reproductive organs lend very little support to the idea that the transplantation of fetal reproductive organs will prove easy or even possible.

Even less is known about the ability of fetal ovaries to function once they are removed from a body. A woman who wanted fetal eggs might have to be present at the abortion clinic and ready for the transplantation of fetal ovarian tissue as soon as an abortion had been performed. This prospect may in itself be sufficient to dampen any interest in the use of fetal gametes.

Even if the technical difficulties with fetal ovarian transplants could be overcome, serious ethical minefields still confront those who want to see this form of transplant tried. Is it really a good idea to allow sperm, eggs, or embryos to be used without the consent of the person to whom they belong? Should the law allow someone to be born without the permission of the parent from whom an egg or sperm is obtained?

At least one state court, the Tennesee Supreme Court in its ruling on the Davis case, a custody dispute over frozen embryos being kept in storage at a fertility clinic, held that it would be against public policy to force someone to become a parent against his or her will. This seems like an extraordinarily sound moral rule. Do not allow parenting without the express consent of the person whose sperm, egg, or embryo is to be used. If they cannot consent, then they should not parent. If parenting without consent is a bad idea, then fetuses would obviously be off-limits for harvesting reproductive tissues.

And would it really be in the best interest of a child to be born from the egg of an aborted fetus? Would women from whose fetuses fetal eggs are procured have the right to claim custody over any child that is born via a transplant should they learn the identity of that child? What would the impact be on children to learn that their grandmother aborted their mother but consented to the use of fetal eggs? True, kids adapt to all sorts of circumstances and challenges but one might hope medicine could come up with a better source of eggs than aborted fetuses.

Fetal egg donation is the latest in a series of stunning promissory notes about how science is changing the way babies are made. Just in the past few years grandmothers have given birth to their own grand-children, postmenopausal women have had babies, sperm from dead men has been used to make children, and the first tentative steps toward the creation of human embryo clones were taken. Science is challenging our definitions of mother, father, parent, and child. The definitions are not written in stone and change is always possible. But before we let change arise we need to be sure that no one need worry that they may be used as a parent without their consent and that the children who are created using technology instead of sex will be the better for it.

Tiny Mermaids

The street I live on is Mermaid Lane. It is a name that somehow does not seem to fit with the city I live in—Philadelphia. More than once I have heard a snicker or snort on the other end of a telephone line when providing my street address. For a lot of people their image of Philadelphia is not one in which anything having to do with mermaids plays a prominent role. But the cynics are wrong.

The notion that somehow a human could live under the sea, effortlessly breathing like a fish, is one that has had sufficient pull on the imaginations of enough of the world's greatest artists to produce fantasy fish names even in a hard-nosed urban setting like Philly. But a kind of mermaid has really now come to Philadelphia. Mermen too. They are to be found in a very unexpected place—the neonatal units of the city's hospitals. Philadelphia has become one of the leading centers of research for liquid ventilation.

An astounding report of human beings being kept alive while breathing only liquids appears in the September 12, 1996 issue of the *New England Journal of Medicine*. The mermaids and mermen were in reality ten tiny premature babies who were kept alive by breathing a liquid. They lived without air for as long as three days in intensive care units in Philadelphia, Buffalo, Seattle, and Los Angeles. Liquid ventilation was used in a desperate effort to save them when their tiny malformed lungs could not absorb enough air, even with the help of mechanical ventilators, for them to survive.

For some years scientists and medical researchers have been trying to develop something that would permit a tiny infant to breathe even when its lungs were not fully formed or were badly damaged. Liquid ventilation using a chemical called a perflurorocarbon, a chemical that is especially fond of oxygen, has emerged as a possible answer. In some animal trials fetal sheep have been able to breathe for as long as 30 days with their bodies completely immersed in a batch of this peculiar brew.

The study in the *New England Journal* reports the first tentative efforts to use liquid ventilation in a human being. Infants were chosen because there are few options available for extremely premature infants that can offer them much hope of survival, and because a human fetus spends all of its formative years in the uterus breathing nothing but liquids. It is not until you or I poke our heads out into the big, big world that our way of getting oxygen switches over from a life in the "sea" of our mother's womb to life in the land of Clinton and Gingrich breathing hot air.

Keeping tiny humans alive in liquid long enough for their lungs to work properly is amazing. But the issues raised by liquid ventilation are even more amazing.

If it does become possible to use liquid ventilation as a reliable treatment for newborns, then it may become possible to push the age at which a fetus can be rescued back farther than the 23- to 24-week limit that now constitutes the boundary of what medicine can try to do to save a newborn life. The implications for the debate about abortion are obvious. And, what works in a fetus might also work in an adult. Someday those who suffer from damage to their lungs from industrial accidents or chemical weapons might spend some time in an intensive care unit breathing liquids until their lungs regain function.

Issues of cost and of risk will have to be weighed, but in the future, a new way of breathing may open up new chances at life. That was always the promise mermaids made to those who fell under their spell.

No Deposit, No Return

Imagine that you and your spouse are expecting a baby. You have just had a visit to the doctor and everything looks great for mom and fetus. The doctor said that if mom keeps watching her weight, stays away from alcohol, and continues to exercise, everything about this pregnancy should turn out just fine. You should be happy but you are not. The culprit is a brochure you grabbed just as you were leaving. It made you nervous about whether you can be a good parent if you fail to sign up for a program to freeze and store stem cells from the afterbirth when your baby is born.

The birth of every baby is accompanied by the elimination of the life-support systems that have kept the baby going inside the uterus—the umbilical cord and placenta. The blood in these tissues contains some very special cells, stem cells, which are proficient at making more blood. Stem cells, the brochure says, can now be extracted from the cord and placenta and frozen at a special storage facility.

Private companies have already started placing brochures with just this message in waiting rooms. The usual request is for parents who are interested to give notice at least a month prior to the due date so that the necessary arrangements can be made.

Why would any parent want to freeze stem cells at birth? The companies promoting stem-cell storage say that genetic blood defects, leukemia, and other cancers can be treated using bone marrow transplants. One corporate brochure warns, however, "there is no way to be sure that bone marrow will be there if your child needs it." If your child suddenly needs marrow and there is no suitable donor among your child's immediate relatives, then, you are told, you are fighting odds on the order of 1 in 20,000 to find a donor. Yikes, what responsible parent would want to leave his or her baby fighting astronomical odds like that when confronting cancer?

Some scientists and doctors believe that stem cell transplants will work as well or better than bone marrow transplants to treat diseases. Dozens of these transplants have been performed. Reports on some of these transplants have appeared in leading medical journals. One recruitment brochure states that "early results are promising" and goes on to note that someday stem cell transplants may prove useful in the treatment of breast cancer, AIDS, and sickle-cell anemia.

If you want to buy biological life insurance for your child, the cost is $1,500. You must also pay an additional $75 annual storage fee.

Nowhere does the brochure suggest that it would be ethically irresponsible not to cough up the cash so your child will have stem cells handy if needed someday. But given the anxieties that pervade the thoughts of expectant parents and the optimistic tone of the brochure, you might well feel like an immoral slug if you didn't fork over the dough to protect junior against the prospect, even a very, very remote one, of a fatal illness.

Every parent deserves information about medical services that might help their newborn child. However, given the newness of stem cell transplants, the fact that bone marrow transplants are rarely needed, and the hypersensitivity of expectant parents, even the most low-key advertising seems high-pressured. The ethics of recruiting soon-to-be parents get even stickier when the cost of doing a stem cell transplant, easily tens of thousands of dollars, enters into the equation. Some parents could bank stem cells only to find out later they do not have the money to pay for their child's transplant.

The sale of any kind of insurance depends on the fear of catastrophe. Selling parents on the need for freezing stem cells is no different. However, without more evidence of need and efficacy, the sale of this type of biological life insurance seems premature. The methods used for recruiting customers deserve very tight regulatory scrutiny. Although parents ought be free to protect their children against even long-shot tiny risks, those who want to sell them the means to do so must be held accountable to the highest ethical standards of advertising and recruitment.

Cyber Medicine

Imagine that your infant son or grandson is in a car accident on a rural road. The EMT personnel suspect head trauma. The boy is rushed to a small local hospital nearby. After examining the child, the doctor is unsure about the extent of the injuries the baby may have suffered. She has not encountered many cases of infant trauma. She says she is going to take some X rays and will send the images electronically to a group of more experienced pediatric head injury experts in at a big teaching hospital in a neighboring state.

You breathe a sigh of relief that technology will make it possible for more experienced specialists to get involved in the baby's care. But in some states the doctor is breaking the law if those pictures are sent!

If you live in Kansas, Texas, Oklahoma, South Dakota, or Nevada, state laws now make it a crime to get second opinions based on images sent electronically from doctors in another state. Twenty other states are flirting with making the practice of sending electronic data and images across state lines illegal. These laws make little sense. They have more to do with protecting the interests of doctors than patients.

Sending medical information through computers and phone lines is called telemedicine. Some medical centers, including the one where I work, the University of Pennsylvania, are rapidly expanding their ability to receive pictures and data from hospitals and clinics anywhere in the world, analyze them, and quickly return their findings. Technology is opening up a whole new way to practice medicine. It is also lucrative for those hospitals and specialists who can take advantage of it.

Some physicians in fields like radiology are extremely worried about telemedicine. If it is possible to beam X rays, CAT scans, PET scans, and other images all over the world in the blink of an eye, why have local specialists at all?

All of the lobbying at state legislatures for restrictions on telemedicine comes from physicians and hospitals worried about the economic impact electronic medicine will have on their medical practice. Self-interest aside, there are some real issues raised by the emergence of telemedicine.

No one has set any standards for the practice of telemedicine. It is not at all clear if there is an error or negligence in interpreting computerized information sent across a state line, which state's laws and courts would have jurisdiction. And is it always in the patient's interest to have his or her X ray read by someone a thousand miles away who cannot personally discuss the findings with the patient and other health care providers?

These questions are legitimate. But simpleminded bans on telemedicine are not. When state legislators respond to worries about economic dislocation by bans, they are seizing on the wrong remedy. The way to grapple with the economic, social, and human costs of technology in medicine is not by swinging a legislative ax to computers and telephone lines. Patients who can benefit from electronic medicine should have every right to do so.

Rethinking the Cost of War

In 1991 American troops were deployed in Kuwait and Iraq. Many years later I sat in a hotel conference room in Kansas City, Missouri, listening to a veteran of that war describe in poignant terms physical problems he believes he contracted as a result of his service in the Gulf War. I was listening to him in my role as a member of the Presidential Advisory Committee on Gulf War Veterans' Illnesses. Many who served this nation during that time are convinced that their cancers, immunological disorders, chronic fatigue, night sweats, or children's birth defects are the result of the time they spent in Kuwait and Iraq.

There are certainly no shortage of potential causes for the varied symptoms and illnesses sometimes lumped under the catchall term, *Gulf War Syndrome*. Sand storms, flies, biological weapons, oil fires, stress, polluted water, unspent rocket fuel, rare microorganisms, antibiological warfare vaccines and drugs, and chemical vapors from bombed Iraqi storage areas are just a few of the things that might have left some of our soldiers sick.

It is difficult to know precisely what might have happened during that conflict that led to the health complaints that make life miserable for many who were there. Exactly who was exposed to what and under what circumstances is tough to reconstruct. It is clear, however, from what took place in the Gulf that we need to begin to think differently about the dangers and costs of modern warfare.

In today's conflicts American military personnel may well find themselves in exotic climates exposed to unfamiliar environments. The battles they fight involve incredible technologies. Modern military technology permits terrible damage to be done to the enemy while making it possible, under the right circumstances, to experience only a minimal number of battlefield casualties among one's own troops.

Fighting hi-tech wars in strange places comes with a poorly understood potential cost. The fuel, paints, cleaning solutions, and chemicals used to maintain and operate all the modern gizmos and gadgets of warfare may carry risks. The poorly understood environments in which war is waged can harbor dangerous substances whose insidious effects may not be readily apparent. Fanatical opponents may resort to all manner of bioecological warfare with physical and psychological results that are not well understood.

One lesson that must be learned from our experience in the Gulf is that we need to take the long-term health threat of hi-tech combat seriously. In order to know whether our active and reserve soldiers have been exposed to biological or chemical agents, beset by strange microbes or parasites, or sickened by environmental toxins and pollutants a clear picture of their health must exist before they go into the field. The Gulf War also shows that accurate records and sound epidemiological monitoring are essential if the price of war is to be accurately calculated. When troops are sent to keep the peace or to fight in places like Somalia, Haiti, or Bosnia it is just as important to arm them with pencils and record books as with guns. The only way to determine who may have been hurt or injured in modern warfare is to have a clear record of who was exposed to what before, during, and after the actual battles are fought.

Baboons and Bone Marrow

A few years ago doctors from the University of California at San Francisco and the University of Pittsburgh killed a baboon, extracted marrow from its bones, and transplanted it into the body of Jeff Getty. The 38-year-old Getty had AIDS. Baboons do not get AIDS. The idea behind the experiment was to give Getty's failing immune system a boost by trying to replace it with the baboon's cells. Some people were troubled that a baboon was sacrificed in order to try this experiment. Killing a baboon might be justified if either a human life could be saved or a great deal of knowledge obtained. Unfortunately, this ill-conceived experiment will not produce either result.

Getty is an AIDS activist who fought for years for the right to be the first to receive a baboon bone marrow transplant. What could possibly be wrong with letting a dying man take his best shot at beating a fatal disease? In the case of baboon bone marrow transplantation, plenty.

Very little research has been done on bone marrow transplantation in primates. What research has been done shows that it is very hard to successfully transplant marrow across species. It is especially difficult to successfully transplant bone marrow among human beings who are not close biological relatives without killing them. One of the lead researchers on the study, Dr. Susan Illstad, says she has found a new type of blood cell, which she calls a facilitator cell, that should make a cross-species transplant possible. Almost no one else in the community of physicians expert at bone marrow transplantation knows what Illstad is talking about. She has published very little about her discovery. Even if she has found a new cell which would allow her to do something that almost no one else believes can possibly work, the tiny amount of animal work reported in medical journals gives no reason to believe that a transplant of baboon bone marrow will do anything but prove to be an effective way to kill a human being.

Getty knew when he agreed to be a subject that the odds were long and that the baboon marrow could kill him. Still, he wanted to try. His consent was important. But it is not enough. When the Grim Reaper is holding the pen in the subject's hand, a signed informed consent is not enough to justify a dubious experiment.

Not only is the science behind trying a baboon bone marrow transplant in a human subject highly suspect, so is the cost. Because a marrow recipient must stay in the hospital for months, it will cost at least $350,000. Remember, this procedure would not have cured Getty or anyone else of AIDS. If it works it merely would help those with AIDS fight off infections. What is the point of pursuing a treatment which if it worked would require farming and killing thousands of baboons at a cost of at least $350,000 per patient that cannot cure anything?

If chasing long odds at huge expense for questionable results does not convince you that baboon marrow transplants are not a promising strategy for curing AIDS, then consider this—baboons may not get AIDS but they get plenty of other nasty diseases. Even baboons raised under the most hygienic conditions may carry and be able to transmit hundreds of different types of viruses to anyone who gets their marrow. And if they do, the marrow recipient could transmit those viruses to the rest of us.

Jeff Getty should never have gotten his chance. Baboon marrow transplants will almost certainly kill anyone who gets one. Even if they do not they are too impractical, too expensive, and put too many people at risk of unknown viral epidemics. Killing baboons for this kind of research makes no sense.

Hearts and Minds

Thirty-four-year-old Sandra Jensen of Sacramento, California, was no Mickey Mantle. Like Mickey Mantle, Sandra Jensen needed a transplant. Unlike Mickey Mantle, Sandra Jensen was rejected sight unseen as a candidate for transplant surgery. The reason she had such a hard time following in Mantle's footsteps is that Sandra Jensen had Down's syndrome.

Most of us know that people with Down's syndrome have various degrees of mental impairment. They also often have other medical problems, including high blood pressure and life-threatening heart defects. Sandra Jensen's heart is malformed and her high blood pressure is destroying her lungs. If she does not get a heart-lung transplant she will die.

Of all the organs used in transplantation, hearts and lungs are the most scarce. Only 90 heart-lung operations were performed last year. Heart-lung transplants are among the most expensive forms of surgery in modern medicine. The cost of such a procedure will certainly run into the hundreds of thousands of dollars.

Sandra was not as severely intellectually impaired as are some others with Downs. She lived on her own and held a job. She had been known to put up a stink when she felt she was not being treated fairly. She and her mother decided, when rejected outright by Stanford University for a transplant, to try the University of California at San Diego.

After an initial evaluation Sandra was rejected there as well. But a campaign was mounted on her behalf mainly by those in the disabilities movement. Disability groups offered financial support and legal representation. The state of California, despite the fact that it is closing down many health services for the poor, promised to pay for her surgery. Religious leaders and public officials tripped over one another to express their outrage that Sandra was initially turned down.

The medical center at San Diego was in a real bind. Although it is against the law to discriminate on the basis of disability, surgeons know that people with Down's have various complex medical problems that often shorten their lives. The transplant team at San Diego believed that with dozens of potential candidates hoping to get one of the few sets of a heart and lungs that become available each month, they are obligated to take the odds of living a full life seriously. Given the other medical problems such as hypertension associated with Down's, Sandra's disability was not, they said, irrelevant to a decision to accept or reject her as a candidate.

Talk of success is reasonable when trying to distribute scarce organs. The problem is that this is not how access to health care now works in America. The patient's ability to pay, citizenship, and geography play crucial roles in determining who lives and who dies. Medical urgency determines who gets first access to a scarce transplant. Other factors such as age, gender, obesity, and health habits can influence the odds of success but are not always treated in the same way as Down's syndrome by transplant programs.

The moral challenge Sandra Jensen posed is whether our nation should distribute expensive and scarce medical resources simply on the basis of who is likely to benefit the most from getting them. If so, those such as Sandra Jensen may not belong on the transplant waiting list since others may stand a better chance of survival. As Mickey Mantle's shot at a transplant made clear, however, more than the chance for success is in play in deciding who lives and who dies in our health care system.

Seeing Straight on Patents

Dr. Samuel Pallin is an Arizona eye surgeon who is mighty peeved. He is angry because a technique he says he discovered for performing cataract surgery without using stitches is being swiped by his fellow surgeons. Many years ago he persuaded the U.S. Patent Office to issue him a patent on the surgical technique. Now he wants his fellow healers to pay him a few bucks in royalties every time they operate. Since there are about a million cataract surgeries done in America every year, Dr. Pallin stands to make a pretty good chunk of change if he can get his peers to cough up.

Many of his fellow doctors think he is, at best, being silly. Jack Singer, a Vermont eye surgeon who works at the Dartmouth-Hitchcock Medical Center in New Hampshire, is one of the physicians Pallin is suing. Singer says he has been using a technique like Pallin's for years. Moreover, he says, hundreds of surgeons do cataract surgery without stitches using slight variations of the specific surgical technique Dr. Pallin claims he invented.

Most of organized medicine thinks Dr. Pallin is worse then silly. They think his call for the right to own and patent surgical techniques is downright dangerous.

The American Medical Association's Council on Ethical and Judicial affairs issued a blistering statement condemning doctors who try to patent surgical techniques on the grounds that "the patenting of medical procedures may increase the cost of treatment, thereby limiting patients access to procedures." The then president of the AMA, Robert McAfee, said of Dr. Pallin's suit, "The mere thought that a procedure would be secretive or that someone would try to profit from it is abhorrent to most physicians and surgeons."

Well, maybe, but profit and health care have been known to mix in American medicine. There are plenty of doctors who hold patents on all sorts of drugs, devices, and therapies and make plenty of money from them. Keeping cures a secret in order to sell them is the basis upon which most of the pharmaceutical and medical device industry operates.

The real issue and the one that the AMA and Pallin's other critics need to focus on is not the legitimacy of patents and profits in medicine, but whether patenting makes sense in the field of surgery where it is technique rather than a product that doctors want to patent.

One reason surgical innovations seem different from products is that they are based on skill. Unlike drugs and devices, which take a lot of upfront financial investment and risk, figuring out new ways to tie a knot or excise dangerous skin growths do not. Society grants patents to encourage innovation in medicine when the economic cost of failure is large and the front-end start-up costs enormous. Surgical innovation does not fit these conditions.

The other reason for discouraging patents in surgery is that the goal of patents is to get discoveries out to the marketplace quickly. Allowing someone to hold a patent on how to cut out a tumor or a better way to perform a C-section may prevent the technique from being disseminated more quickly. Patients might die because those who hold patents on how to operate will not share their knowledge.

Sam Pallin thinks that he deserves compensation for his surgical discovery. The U.S. Patent Office agrees. But before a court makes his fellow eye surgeons pony up, Congress had better take a long hard look at the issue of whether allowing a surgeon to collect a royalty every time an appendix is removed or a cut stitched is really in your best interest.

Why Say No to Life

The allegations of favoritism that surrounded Mickey Mantle's liver transplant are a powerful reminder that there are far more people waiting for transplants than there are organs to give to them. The question is with so many people dying who might be able to provide organs to those in need, why are there so few organs available for transplant? An important new study sheds some light on this puzzle.

Almost 5,000 people were waiting for liver transplants when Mantle got his. Only 3,500 liver transplants were performed in all of 1994. Since more than 25,000 people die each year from liver failure, the list of those waiting could be even longer if there were more organs to use. The same dismal story of people dying for want of organs can be told about the tens of thousands of Americans currently awaiting kidney, pancreas, heart, or lung transplants.

The largest source of organs for transplantation come from those who are declared brain-dead while on life-supporting technologies. While estimates are that anywhere from 6,000 to 10,000 people might die under circumstances that would permit them to be used as organ donors, the number of organs actually obtained is far below even the low end of this estimate. Why?

A team of researchers at the University of Pittsburgh led by Laura Siminoff and Robert Arnold, Beth Virnig now of the University of Miami, and I published the findings of a two-year study in the *Annals of Internal Medicine* which provides the answer. The reason is simple but dismaying. Many families simply do not give their consent when asked for organ donation.

We found that, although the possibility of organ donation was relatively rare, nearly every case where someone might have been a donor was identified by someone in the hospital where the person died. Moreover, laws requiring inquries to be made about donation are being followed. Most families were asked. Sadly, however, only 48 percent of those asked said yes. The percentage of those willing to permit tissue donation such as skin, bones, or corneas was far lower.

These numbers are startling because opinion polls conducted by many organizations and polling groups over the years have shown widespread public support for organ donation and transplantation.

Some surveys report that 60 to 70 percent of those asked say they would donate their organs or allow donation from a deceased relative. So where is all this apparent altruism when it is needed most?

The reasons families object hinge on a lack of faith and trust. Many families express religious reservations about organ donation. Some talk about their fears about harming the deceased or mutilating the body of their loved one. Some simply do not trust the medical system, worrying that relatives will be allowed to die prematurely if permission to donate is given, are ambivalent due to the belief that there are gross inequities in how organs are used to save lives, or are just angry at what they perceive to be insensitive requests.

Some people have argued that what we need to do to get more organs and tissues for transplant is to create a market in body parts. Others maintain that we should pass laws presuming that individuals consent to donation and put the burden on those who are opposed to carry a card or inform their relatives.

Our study shows that neither of these approaches will work. The most important reason people do not donate has nothing to do with money or with selfishness. They do not donate because they find the subject distasteful, they feel their religious beliefs will be compromised, they are not asked in a respectful manner, or they do not believe the system is fair. Until these problems are resolved the gap between those who need a transplant to live and those who take their organs with them to the grave will never be bridged.

Breast Cancer and BMT

Throughout the country there are insurance companies that refuse to pay for medical treatment for women with advanced-stage breast cancer. They seem to be robbing some women of their last hope for life. The state of Minnesota is one state that wrestled with legislation that might change this situation for its residents. A bill was passed that requires insurance companies to cover the costs of high-dose chemotherapy in combination with bone marrow transplantation for women with breast cancer. The Minnesota law seems like a good idea. It may not be.

High-dose chemotherapy with bone marrow transplantation is a new way to battle some forms of breast cancer. When the cancer has spread, doctors can try a last-ditch attack. They remove and store special cells called stem cells from the patient's body. The doctors, knowing the stem cells have been stored, can then try to use much higher doses of chemotherapy than are usually tried to attack the cancer cells. Even if they do terrible damage to the woman's immune system by aggressively going after the cancer, they can try to repair things by using a bone marrow transplant to put back the stored stem cells.

High-dose chemotherapy with bone marrow transplantation is expensive. It can cost anywhere from $50,000 to $200,000.

And the number of women who might want to try this procedure is large. There will be more than 182,000 new cases of breast cancer diagnosed in the United States this year. While some progress is being made in treating breast cancer, almost 50,000 Americans will die this year from the disease.

Politicians, some experts in the field of breast cancer, and some women's advocacy groups have argued that the only humane and decent thing to do is to give those facing the grim diagnosis of terminal breast cancer a chance by requiring insurers to pay the tab. Many courts in a number of states have ordered insurers to pay for the treatment. Four states besides Minnesota—Massachusetts, Virginia, New Hampshire, and Vermont—have enacted legislation requiring insurance companies and medical plans to provide coverage. The federal government in 1996 began requiring coverage for all nine million federal employees and their dependents. So why shouldn't other states require coverage too?

According to a study by Pennsylvania-based ECRI, a widely respected nonprofit agency that does assessments of new medical technologies and treatments, there is no evidence that high-dose chemotherapy in combination with bone marrow transplantation works. What is worse, the treatment might actually shorten the lives of some of those who receive it.

ECRI looked at all available studies reported in the medical literature of high-dose chemotherapy in combination with breast cancer and found no evidence "of any prolonged disease-free or overall survival benefit" in women who had this treatment as opposed to standard care and substantial evidence of decreased ". . . survival time and one year overall survival." If the ECRI study is right, high-dose chemotherapy with bone marrow transplantation, while touted by some as a last best slim hope, does not work and might make some women even sicker.

When facing a dread disease our most common reaction is to suppose that doing something, anything, is better than doing nothing. But as the ECRI study shows, that is not always true. For now women with breast cancer who want to receive high-dose chemotherapy with bone marrow transplantation must be fully informed about what is known and not known. The procedure should only be done in carefully designed research trials so that its efficacy can be determined with more certainty. As unlikely as it seems, it is possible that the most humane choice insurers could make is to do nothing.

Laser Blinding

Did Harry Truman do the right thing in ordering two atomic bombs to be dropped on Japanese cities at the end of World War II? An exhibit at the Smithsonian museum in Washington, D.C., added fuel to an already red-hot debate about the morality of using the atomic bomb. Debates about the morality of developing and using weapons capable of causing great harm seem somehow to belong to our past. Not so. Technological advances in laser weaponry give special significance to our willingness to assess what happened to Hiroshima and Nagasaki five decades ago.

Originally the Smithsonian exhibit raised some tough and contentious questions about whether our leaders made the right decision in using a weapon that killed 140,000 civilians, including many women and children. But veterans groups such as the American Legion and the Air Force Association demanded a copy of the text that was going to accompany the Enola Gay exhibit. They were angry at what they saw. Those who survived the carnage of places such as Iwo Jima and Pearl Harbor thought the planned Smithsonian exhibit did not adequately address the political and military considerations that led Truman to order the use of the bomb.

The skeptical tone of the exhibit was toned down as a result of the directive by the then head of the Smithsonian, I. Michael Heyman. But the moral questions raised by the invention of weapons of mass destruction do not end at the door of a museum.

Scientists have been at work for some time now on a new weapon—laser blinding. Lasers capable of the mass blinding of soldiers and civilians will soon become a part of the arsenals of many nations unless outlawed by international treaty.

A laser using the same wavelength as visible light can be constructed which can focus on the retina of the eye. This causes the blood vessels in the eye to be destroyed, resulting in nearly instantaneous and complete blinding. Treatment is impossible.

The lasers capable of wreaking this sort of havoc are small and highly portable. They can be carried like a large rifle with a small battery pack in a harness to provide energy. They are completely silent. All one needs to do is to get the target to look at the device, even from hundreds of yards away, and their sight will be forever lost.

Even in war, much less self-defense, the international community has agreed that some weapons are too cruel, too malignant to use. Dumdum bullets, gas, land mines and biological weapons have all been banned under various international agreements including the United Nations Convention on Certain Conventional Weapons.

Is the ability to suddenly and permanently blind your enemy so gruesome and cruel that this form of weaponry ought to be added to the list of prohibited weapons? Or should we keep this weapon in our arsenal, remembering that 50 years ago the leaders of this nation decided to use another deadly weapon.

According to the British medical journal *The Lancet*, the cost of mass blinding would be enormous. Coping with thousands, perhaps hundreds of thousands, of blind soldiers and civilians, laser weapons would cost more than most societies could bear.

Even if it was a morally defensible choice, there should be no debate that questioning why it was right to use the atomic bomb requires no defense. In examining and explaining the decision made 50 years ago we may see more clearly the answer to whether it is right to construct weapons that blind instantly today.

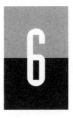

Rationing Cost

Did the Mick Get A Break?

By all accounts Mickey Mantle was one hell of a baseball player. By all accounts Mickey Mantle was also one hell of a hell-raiser. Both aspects of his life intersected in an operating room in Dallas, Texas, when Mantle received a liver transplant to repair the one he had destroyed through decades of alcohol abuse. Even before Mantle got out of the operating room questions were raised about the ethics of his surgery. Primary among them was the opinion that a jerk who wrecks his body does not deserve a liver.

Excluding sinners from medical care would greatly reduce medical costs. No one would be in the hospital except a few newborn babies and some elderly persons who formerly dwelled in monastaries. If Mickey Mantle did not deserve a liver because he spent many years as a drunk, does Christopher Reeve deserve care for his damaged spinal cord which he brought on himself by his chosen hobby of riding a horse? And after we're done croaking Mantle and Reeve for their sins should we then throw everyone out of the hospital who is there because they smoked, drank, chewed tobacco, had sex without protection, did not wear a helmet or seatbelt, drove a car too fast, had an accident while hunting, slipped getting into their hot tub, fell rock climbing, lopped off a body part operating a combine, snow blower, ax, or lawn mower, went over the handlebars of their bicycle, overate, attempted suicide, took drugs, worked in a high-stress job, or got hurt playing high school, college, or pro sports? Let's face it, hospitals are for sinners and there are plenty of us.

More curious was the short time that elapsed between the time Mr. Mantle was listed as needing a liver transplant and the surgery. This turn of events left the nation dumbstruck. Is it possible, experts and pundits inquired, that someone who is famous, wealthy, or both could have access to life-saving medical resources that other less blessed occupants of these 50 states might enjoy? One must presume these souls slept peacefully through the debate about reforming this nation's flawed health care system.

Did it help to be Mickey Mantle to get a transplant? Well, how many other 63-year-old-men with cirrhosis of the liver, hepatitis, liver cancer, and relatively little money have received liver transplants in recent years? A generous estimate could include zero in its range and not be too far off.

The transplant community, upon hearing doubts that the system plays fair, harrumphed and protested in solemn tones that in the distribution of vital inner parts obtained from the newly deceased, equity and justice are the only thoughts that flit through medical minds. And to some extent that is true. Once on a waiting list, the criteria used to decide who gets the next available liver are almost exclusively biological. Once on the waiting list, Mickey Mantle did not have to push anyone else out of the operating room to get his liver. But, the sole reason he was on the waiting list is that he was Mickey Mantle.

Money is the crucial element determining who makes it through a hospital's door when an expensive form of treatment is needed. If you do not have money or insurance, then celebrity will do since this will either help you get money or will attract attention to the medical center if they supply you free care. If you need a $300,000 procedure and lack health insurance, as 25 million or more Americans do, bring money or at least become notorious before you head for the hospital.

Mickey Mantle probably will not be remembered as a crusader for health care reform. But the fact that the baseball legend gained access to a liver transplant points out flaws so profound and fundamental in our health care system they ought not continue to be ignored.

Who Goes First?

When Mickey Mantle received his liver transplant howls of protest went up across the nation. It was no secret that his liver failure was a direct result of his days spent carousing as a young ballplayer. How could the Mick latch on to a transplant when so many other, more "worthy," potential recipients, could not?

The United Network for Organ Sharing, the group responsible for setting allocation policies for access to liver and other forms of transplants in the United States, has taken a bold step toward insuring fair access to liver transplants. Officials of the Richmond, Virginia, based UNOS announced at their annual meeting in Boston in December, 1996 that, patients who stand the best chance of surviving a transplant and living longer will get preference over those waiting for livers. That means that people who are otherwise healthy who suffer sudden unexpected liver failure (e.g., from eating a poisonous mushroom) and children would move to the head of the liver line.

Mickey Mantle would not have had the same shot at a transplant under the new UNOS rules. Howls of protest greeted the announcement.

The complaints came from those on the liver waiting list suffering from chronic liver failure often due to alcohol abuse, and transplant centers with many such patients. They were not happy at the prospect of even a slight move down in priority, for livers are so scarce that a lower priority may well mean no transplant at all.

The outrage of those likely to move lower on the waiting list is understandable. The issue of who goes first on the waiting list is not a matter of ethical theory for someone dying of liver failure. From the point of view of the individual patient, the only fair policy is the one that gets them a liver.

However, that is not what is fair from the point of view of those who need to allocate livers to all persons in need. Their duty is to try and get the most good from the limited resource they have available.

Some of those hurt by the decision to give greater priority to relatively healthy patients and children say that the decision represents bias against those whose livers no longer function as a result of heavy drinking. Not so.

The fact is sin and personal worth have nothing to do with the shift in UNOS policy toward patients who are the most likely to benefit from a $200,000 liver transplant. If the goal of liver transplantation is to save lives, then the morally just policy is to use the scarce supply of livers not to help those who have waited the longest or who have been sick the longest, but to those most likely to live.

Assigning priority to those on transplant waiting lists who are getting sicker and sicker while they wait at death's door is not the most efficient or effective way to save lives. UNOS was right to try to shift allocation policies to reflect the best available knowledge about who can benefit the most from access to a transplant. That is not bias or prejudice, it is simply the best solution to a tragic choice.

Bad Apples

Bartolome Moya is not the sort of fellow you would want to meet in a dark alley. The 37-year-old Moya has been accused by federal authorities of multiple murders, kidnappings, bombings, impersonating a police officer, and racketeering. Officials at the Department of Justice are convinced that Moya was, until recently, the kingpin of an incredibly malicious New York City drug ring.

You may think that Moya is a man who does not deserve much pity or compassion from society. You are right. But Moya was shown a great deal of compassion by doctors at Temple University Medical Center in Philadelphia. Despite Moya's alleged record of brutal crimes and cruel violence, they were right to do so.

In August of 1993, Moya and some of the alleged members of his gang were indicted by a federal grand jury in Manhattan. Three of Moya's co-defendants were convicted and sentenced to life in prison without parole. However, Moya fell ill during the trial. When examined by a court-appointed medical team, he was diagnosed as having terminal heart disease.

Mr. Moya was given only a few months to live. Thomas Griesa, then chief judge of Federal Court in Manhattan, released him from the trial to spend his final days with his family who had just moved to Philadelphia. Moya joined them, but early in 1994 he also signed up for the heart transplant waiting list at Temple.

Many who wait for heart transplant die before they even get a chance at surgery. Only about one in three adults awaiting a heart transplant actually gets a new lease on life. Moya was one of the lucky few.

On February 24, a heart became available in Philadelphia for which Moya was the best possible recipient on biological grounds. Since his doctors had no idea that he had a rap sheet a mile long, they did not hesitate to transplant him. Public funds paid for his transplant to the tune of $400,000. In fact not only did Moya get an expensive form of life-saving therapy free, he used the transplant to evade subsequent efforts by the feds to renew his prosecution.

In July, federal marshals reindicted the recuperating Moya and put him under house arrest in Philadelphia. Aware that his odds of heading to prison were very, very good, he jumped his $250,000 bail and, on July 19, disappeared. On October 22, police in Santo Domingo in the Dominican Republic, working with U.S. marshals, found and arrested him. He appeared to be in very good health.

Moya's ability to wangle a transplant out of the doctors at Temple at public expense has led to a great deal of public outcry. Television programs, op-ed writers, radio blab-meisters, and editorialists have wondered how a man who appears to be nothing less then a brutal criminal can wriggle his way to get very expensive transplant surgery at public expense. Most of the outrage has focused on the doctors at Temple who many say did not do enough to investigate the seamy background of their patient. The critics of the doctors are wrong.

Health care professionals, whether they are transplant surgeons or other sorts of specialists, are in the business of healing not punishing. They have no right to assess the moral worth of those who need their services. Doctors have no special training or skill to bring to bear to decide who has sinned too much to merit care. And unless you yourself are free from vice, it might not be a good idea to advocate a system in which doctors apply culpability and morality tests before deciding whether you merit medical care.

If society does not want Bartolome Moyas on its transplant lists, it must pass the requisite legislation to keep criminals from gaining entry. There is no excuse for blaming medicine when the answer to the question of whether criminals should be eligible for transplants ought to be found in our statehouses not our hospitals.

Race and Medicine

Americans are obsessed with race. Every aspect of life in these United States, from housing to education, from immigration to welfare, is permeated by attention to race. From the relentless attention given the trial of O. J. Simpson to the growing chorus of calls for an end to affirmative action, race is never gone from our thoughts for long.

American medicine is no different; it is also obsessed with race. When doctors present cases for discussion with their colleagues, the first sentence they utter always provides the race of the patient. When doctors and public health officials report data on how effective certain treatments are in the battle against disease and disability, those numbers are almost always broken out on the basis of race. When government agencies talk about problems of health insurance coverage or access to health care, race is the single most important category used to analyze the state of the American health care system.

Obviously race does sometimes matter in medicine. The identification of patients sometimes requires information about their race or ethnicity. And there are certain diseases such as sickle-cell, cystic fibrosis, spina bifida, and Tay-Sachs where race or ethnicity may make a difference in trying to arrive at a diagnosis. But American medicine, like American society in general, often pays too much attention to race despite the fact that racial categories frequently serve no real purpose or actually obscure more important facts.

Stephen Caldwall and Rebecca Popenoe of the University of Virginia argue in the April 15, 1996 issue of the *Annals of Internal Medicine* that the crude categories "black" and "white" or "Asian," which are used to identify patients are just that—crude. They contend that using these terms may actually obscure important facts about biological or behavioral differences among individuals that a doctor needs to know to make the right diagnosis or arrive at the best treatment. Calling everyone from a fourth-generation Norwegian American to a recent Jewish immigrant from Iraq white may obscure cultural or biological differences that really matter to health. Lumping everyone into a few generic racial categories obscures the fact that it is sometimes the differences among those in a category rather than differences between them that are important for diagnosis and treatment.

Christopher Bagley, writing in the April, 1996 issue of *Social Science and Medicine*, also makes a plea for less overt racism in medicine. He notes that by collecting data on treatment outcomes and mortality on the basis of race there is a very real danger of overlooking the most important factor that determines your health—money.

Americans are used to hearing that blacks do not fare as well as whites in getting treatment for cancer or hypertension. Every year statistical reports are issued showing that there are more premature births among blacks then whites. But these racial classifications obscure the fact that what really counts in determining whether you get prenatal care or give birth to a premature baby is not the color of your skin but how much money is in your pocket.

Because Americans are more comfortable with racial divisions than economic ones, the problems of our health care system are often put in terms of black and white. But as any poor uninsured person can tell you, green is the color that really counts when your health is on the line.

Affording Our Miracles

Ivy Hill Cemetery is located in Philadelphia not far from where I live. Just before Christmas in 1996, 24-year-old Lolita Cunningham was buried there. Relatively few people outside her immediate family noticed. Twelve years made quite a difference in her ability to get others to pay attention to her.

In 1985, when she became Philadelphia's first child to receive a heart transplant, everyone cared what happened to Lolita Cunningham. The most advanced resources medicine had to offer were brought to bear to save her life. Money was not an issue. By 1996, money had become an issue and the health care system had allowed her to flounder. Her death reveals a lot about what is wrong with our health care system, a system that makes enormous efforts to rescue people from death's door but has no time for those who are merely hanging around in the waiting room.

Lolita was born with a deformed heart. It kept her alive for a while but, as she grew, it could no longer support her body. Doctors at St. Christopher's Hospital for Children in Philadelphia decided to risk a heart transplant. It worked.

Lolita did very well after the transplant. She kept up her health by carefully following the strict regimen of expensive medication to which all heart transplant recipients must adhere. Although her family was very poor, she managed to stay in school. Eventually she was admitted to Philadelphia's Drexel University. Even though money problems forced her to drop out, she was able, with the university's help, to land a job as a part-time lab assistant at SmithKline Beecham Corporation. She used her pay to get her own apartment. But despite overcoming the handicap of a failing heart, Lolita could not overcome a health care system that all too often lets people fall through financial and social cracks.

Her foster mom, Brenda Datts, says Lolita became angry and depressed when, after getting a job, she lost her eligibility for Medicaid assistance. Without this coverage it became very hard for her to pay the $600 a month for the drugs that keep a transplanted heart working. Lolita Cunningham became one of millions of Americans who, because they are part-time employees, do not qualify for health insurance through their jobs.

Datts says, that because of worries about cost, her daughter stopped going to the doctor for her regular checkups. And as her worries about money and insurance grew she began to skip her medications. Without her medicine her transplanted heart could not function. In the summer of 1996 she wound up in a hospital emergency room at Temple University Medical Center. Her bills kept mounting. And her depression about her financial problems and her concern that she was becoming a burden to others did too.

Lolita Cunningham kept playing Russian roulette with her medicine. Just before Christmas she lost. She called her mom from her job to complain that she was not feeling well. Her mom said she should go right to the hospital. She said she "didn't want to bother anybody." Less then an hour later an ambulance had to be called. Less than a day later she died.

A health care system that knew no boundaries when a little girl's life was on the line had no room for a 24-year-old woman trying to make her own way in the world. A society that prides itself on going all out to rescue the dying is indifferent to the health care needs of those with chronic problems. And a health care system that can move hearts from the dead to the living has no room in its heart for the depressed and despondent. Lolita Cunningham deserved better from all of us.

Home Health Fraud

I know it is tiresome. I sympathize with your unwillingness to read one more word about government ineptitude. No need to tell me I am trying your patience in asking you to continue to peruse this space knowing that all you will get is irritated. Still, the gargantuan fraud that is Medicare coverage for home health care demands your attention.

By most estimates fraud accounts for nearly 10 percent of all the money spent on Medicare. Talk about the impending bankruptcy of federal health programs for the elderly and the poor is everywhere. Many in Congress fascinated with tearing Medicare to shreds refuse to do anything about the hemorrhaging of funds into the hands of crooks wearing white coats and their avaricious business partners. The latest evidence of the bonanza that corporate crooks enjoy at your expense is to be found in a new General Accounting Office report whose title says it all: "Home Health Utilization Expands While Program Controls Deteriorate." It is grim reading.

Providing care such as medical evaluations, skilled nursing services, physical therapy, speech therapy, and medical social services to older Americans in their homes seems like a good idea. It allows your grandparents to stay in familiar surroundings and to maintain their habits and lifestyles. One might suppose that care given in the home would be cheaper than that provided in a hospital. But if the program that pays people to provide these services lacks basic financial controls, oversight, and accountability, no one should be surprised that it is rife with rip-offs, scams, and fraud. As a result, home care paid for under Medicare is a pretty expensive proposition.

In 1989, 1.7 million Medicare beneficiaries received home health care services. In 1993, the last year for which figures are available, 2.8 million were getting care at home. But here comes an astounding number: Medicare spent $2.7 billion on home health care in 1989. In 1993 it spent $11 billion! More than four times as much money was spent on not even double the number of people between 1989 and 1993.

Why the boom? The GAO says that the 1993 beneficiaries are not sicker or more frail then they were in 1989. However, each person in the program it charges, submitted twice as many billable visits as they did four years ago. Oh, did I mention that the number of organizations in the Medicare home health care business stood at 5,692 in 1989 and that there were more than 7,500 of them by 1993? Notably 80 percent of the new entrants into the home health care field are private, for-profit agencies. Greedy entrepreneurs have realized that the federal government has no ability to monitor claims, bills, or conduct audits to see whether anyone charging for home care is actually doing anything.

The GAO notes that in the face of this bonanza for the unscrupulous, Congress, in the name of deregulation, has actually cut the budget for regulatory oversight and audits of claims in Medicare in half. So even though every dollar spent on regulating Medicare claims for home health care returns $14 by detecting phony charges, ineligible recipients, and fraudulent service scams, the home health care benefit in Medicare remains a spigot of easy profits. For those willing to dip into your tax dollars allegedly to provide good care to your parents and grandparents, Congress has made sure there is no place like home.

Newt and Gruel

The newspapers and television are full of Newt. America has no choice. If you turn on your TV or pick up a paper or magazine it is either going to be the embers of the O.J. circus or Newt Gingrich yammering on about how proud and satisfied he is with the job he is doing. Wherever Newt gambols in media land he dispenses his self-congratulatory report card. Incredibly almost no one, including who-ever it is that currently occupies the large white building on Pennsylvania Avenue, seems willing to take him to task for his arro-gance and indifference to how poorly government is really doing in meeting the needs of all its citizens. O.J. might get away with it. Newt ought not. It would not be fair to the abused and mentally ill kids who live a few streets away from where Newt works in the kid's ward at St. Elizabeth's psychiatric hospital to let his blarney pass unnoticed.

St. Elizabeth's is a sprawling facility for the mentally ill located almost in the shadow of Capitol Hill. It took in its first patient in 1855. Founded by social reformer and mental health pioneer Dorothea Dix, the institution adhered to a view that was novel for its day and, is sadly, if one takes Newt seriously, novel in ours. Dix argued that if we treat the mentally ill kindly and with dignity, some might recover. Newt ought to take a few minutes out from hobnobbing with publish-ing magnates and $5,000-a-plate dinners and drop in on the 12-and-under-patients at St. Elizabeth's. They see the impact of welfare cuts in a somewhat different light than Newt.

On March 13, 1995, there was a food riot at St. Elizabeth's. Fifty mentally ill kids, many between five and ten, started acting up after finding out all they were going to get to eat that day was rice, gravy, and Jell-O. They had received the same for the past three weeks. In-spectors from the Public Health Service have subsequently confirmed that mentally ill kids under 12, most on large doses of psychiatric drugs, have been given nothing but rice and Jell-O with a few bits of meat for many weeks. No fruit, no vegetables, and nothing else has been served because St. Elizabeth's is broke. The city of Washington's mental health commissioner, Guido Zanni, said the hospital had no money to buy food.

Handwringing about the fate of the disadvantaged poor is not popular at this time in American history. The backlash that Newt and his ilk rode to power was fueled by the perception that "we" have done enough for "them" and that it is "our" turn to get what "we" are due.

But should Newt really be allowed to wander around from television studio to radio microphone braying to his fellow citizens that he is proud of what he has done in office while 50 mentally ill kids are living right down the road on gravy and Jell-O? What is the moral credibility of a social revolution that leaves mentally ill and abused kids with little to eat?

The key measure of Newt's leadership and that of the current Congress should be what is on the plate at St. Elizabeth's. In fact it might be a good idea to insist that the same trucks that deliver paltry meals to St. Elizabeth's youngest residents deliver precisely the same food to the House and Senate dining rooms. A few weeks on the St. Elizabeth's diet would do politicians a world of good.

Pick On Someone Your Own Size

A few years ago Phyllis Kahn, a Minnesota state legislator, proposed granting children the right to vote. The idea was hooted down as ridiculous. When you look at the willingness of Congress to balance the federal budget on the small shoulders of kids, you have to wonder.

If kids could vote they might be able to protect themselves against a Republican plan to trim the bloated federal budget by making it harder for them to see a doctor. By turning the Medicaid program into a state-run program where the federal government simply gives out block grants with no eligibility or coverage requirements, millions of kids could wind up with no health insurance.

Congress has already dealt kids a bad hand when it comes to health care. More than nine million American children have no health insurance. The number of Americans without health insurance is growing fastest among the children of the working poor.

More and more moms and dads work in businesses that, because of escalating health care costs, do not offer any health insurance at all or do not include coverage for dependents. The only hope kids in these situations have to get health insurance is Medicaid. The federal government requires every state to provide limited insurance coverage to the children of poor families.

Medicaid is a prime target of congressional budget balancers. The cost of the program has been increasing for years. It is projected to rise from $131 billion to $260 billion over the next five years. But kids are not the reason why.

The reason for Medicaid's escalating costs is that increasing numbers of Americans are living longer and longer. Some of these people require expensive nursing home care and home care. But because Medicare does not pay for these services, more and more older Americans are shuffling around their assets in order to impoverish themselves so Medicaid picks up the tab. But Congress prefers not to wrestle with groups that can vote. By talking about block grants that would do away with minimal federal mandates to cover children, Congress can quietly put the screws to the group of Americans least able to defend itself at the ballot box. Without federal pressure many states facing their own budget crises will continue to restrict or drop health insurance coverage for kids, especially for those whose parents work.

Only a bunch of blockheads could come up with a plan which would turn Medicaid into a no-strings-attached handout program for the states. When it comes to divvying up the burdens of balancing the budget, kids should carry the least of the load. Congress should stop bullying children with Medicaid cuts. They should pick on those who at least have the power to throw them out of office.

Medicaid Fraud

The governor of Pennsylvania, Tom Ridge, must be pretty handy with an ax. There is no other way to explain why he and the legislators in the state House and Senate are the latest in a growing list of public officials throughout the country enthusiastically hacking away at the health of the poor to save money. Governor Ridge has cut Medicaid coverage for more than 260,000 Pennsylvanians. Balancing budgets by lopping the poor out of state sponsored health care make no sense.

Before the ax falls those who wield it must be prepared to say why they have no choice. True, Medicaid is one of the biggest expenditures that state governments face. But why? This is a question hackers like Governor Ridge seem unable and even unwilling to answer.

One reason Medicaid costs so much is that it has been allowed to become a welfare program for the middle and upper classes. Since this nation has no program to pay for long-term and nursing home care for elderly Americans (costs not covered by Medicare), Medicaid has become the way to go. Every state's Medicaid program, including Pennsylvania's, is chock full of elderly folks who transferred or spent down their assets so as to appear poor in order to qualify for Medicaid. There is a coven of lawyers and accountants who do nothing more for a living than think up ways for the wealthy to transfer their assets so as to avoid getting stuck with the high cost of nursing home care. Governor Ridge and his likeminded legislative cronies across the nation have done little to stop this scam. Much easier to boldly wield the budgetary ax against children, single head of household women, and the working poor for whom Medicaid was originally intended than to take on the subsidies of the middle class.

What is completely senseless about making cuts in Medicaid is that somebody is going to pay when the poor get sick. Since we have not yet adopted the practice of leaving the victims of car accidents, strokes, muggings, and industrial accidents to die where they lay, they will still get taken to hospitals. And, doctors and nurses will treat them. The only question then is who will get stuck with the tab for their bills? Will it be Congress, the state legislature, the city, the county, or the treating hospital? Proposals to saw off the Medicaid limb for the poor are really nothing more than a giant shell game whose only rationale is to pass the cost on to somebody else.

Throwing people out of Medicaid is both dumb and unethical. It fails to keep people healthy and it simply leaves those who care for the poor with the job of finding somebody else to stick with the bill. The nation's governors and state legislators must do better. They need to examine why Medicaid costs as much as it does before attacking it with meat-cleaver solutions. Medicaid's woes are merely symptomatic of our society's failure to provide help in paying for long-term care for those who need it and to reform what is a broken, fractured, and dying non-system of health insurance.

The Price of Mainstreaming

Sometimes the price of being fair is high. Once in awhile it is so high that it becomes unfair. That is what has happened as a result of America's desire to make sure that kids with severe disabilities get an equal chance at an education.

Not too long ago I visited an elementary school in a suburb of Minneapolis. A friend of mine had a child in the second grade. He had picked me up to take me to a meeting and on the way we stopped to pick up his son from school. We walked into the classroom where I could not help but notice a small boy in a bed surrounded by monitors and some other medical paraphernalia.

The boy lay absolutely still. There was a nurse sitting nearby reading. I thought the boy was asleep. I half-jokingly asked the teacher if all her students fell asleep in class. She looked at me with a very sad expression and said that the boy was not asleep. He was in a coma and she was certain he had never been awake in the five months he had been brought to her class.

Why was a comatose boy being brought to school? Because, the teacher explained, his parents thought that maybe he could still perceive despite the coma and they wanted him in a regular classroom.

I had put this incident out of my mind until I happened to read a story by Dante Chinni in *The Washington Monthly*. Chinni found that as a result of the Individuals with Disabilities Education Act, which Congress passed and then-President Ford signed in 1975, school districts all around the nation are burdened with huge expenses as a result of their legal obligation to provide educational services to kids with severe disabilities. School districts in New York, Virginia, California, New Jersey, and many other states are paying hundreds of thousands of dollars per year to educate a single child with a severe disability. In South Portland, Maine, Chinni found, the public schools must deal with a bill of more than $120,000 per year to cover the costs of educating four children with severe autism.

Every child deserves an education, even an expensive one in the case of a child with a disability. But at some point providing education for a few begins to infringe on the rights of too many others.

Congress should take another look at what its 20-year-old underfunded mandate is doing to our public schools. Caps should be set on what a school district must pay to educate a child. There should be more cost sharing between state, federal, and local authorities. Affluent families with a disabled child should not have the right to the same subsidies as do the children of poor families.

A moral community owes its frail and weakest members a fair shot at fulfilling their potential. But when the price of educating a single child becomes so great that it threatens a community's ability to educate the rest of its kids, it is time to think about the limits of community duty. When a child in a coma is attending public school, it is time to think harder about what is real and what is symbolic in the efforts to provide equal opportunity to all regardless of disability.

Why Must I Live So Long?

Could the news be any worse? As is their usual custom, TV, radio, and the newspapers repeated it incessantly. No surprise there. The media are always wallowing in human misery. Perhaps you do not know what I am talking about because you tuned out since you could not take one more bit of evidence that things are worse than they appear. You might want to stop reading right now for I fear I have no choice but to transmit the grim news.

Okay, you're still with me so don't say I didn't give you fair warning. Here goes: death rates from cancer are falling in this country. As many as 16,000 Americans will survive cancer this year who would have died in 1990. Sorry to ruin your breakfast. I know, I know, it is hard to imagine anything more depressing.

Excuse me? Did I hear someone whisper that it really might not be such a bad thing if more people live longer? Duh. Well, hey, don't be expecting a job as a congressional staffer, White House fellow, think-tank policy wonk, or newspaper pundit anytime soon. If you don't see that more people living longer is a tragedy, then you are truly clueless.

Sure, sure, generations before us would have given all their wealth and possessions to achieve what we enjoy in terms of a chance at a long life. An American of George Washington's day would say that there could be no better proof that the descendants of this nation's founders had gone stark raving nuts than to find today's citizenry beset with communal despair over the fact they are living longer. But that is why I am the professor and you, with your limited ability to grasp the big picture, are not.

Remember our primitive forbears lived in an age when there were no supplemental retirement account executives, Council of Economic Advisors, and health benefits plan managers. If they had had these doyens they would have known that a fate in which lots of folks make it to old age is to be feared and dreaded.

True, when you talk to particular people about growing old, almost no one says that want a short lifespan for themselves. But that is precisely why trendy, shallow group-thinking is needed. Taken as a vague, amorphous whole, old age looks awful. Looked at as a group, grandmothers become geezers and your duties to parents become backbreaking burdens on the next generation.

Only snivelers, weenies, and she-men would worry that the old deserve respect and dignity. Only a person with tunnel vision would fail to see that living longer means that you are only postponing the inevitable and what is the point of that? What the elderly deserve is not to suck the lifeblood out of the rest of society with their wastrel ways and spendthrift habits.

The reason living longer is no good is because it costs too much. Old people, as any dour economist can tell you, require lots of resources. The older you are the greater your need is for special housing, an income, and medical care. Laughably, there are some among us who think that just because they are old they are entitled to dip their liver-spotted hands into your wallet.

What is worse, our grimmest future forecasters tell us, it did not have to be this way. If today's baby boomers hadn't been so busy in their most fertile years listening to the Beatles and Stones, inhaling marijuana, dodging military service, swallowing birth control pills, bumming around Europe, wallowing in the mud at Woodstock, and otherwise frittering away their best procreative years, they would have spawned enough offspring to support them in the style to which they will want to become accustomed as they dodder into old age. The only person you will have to blame when you survive your bout of cancer and wind up still on the planet at age 80 is Timothy Leary and he managed to scram out of here before anyone could call him to account.

Enough irony. It makes for lousy domestic policy. It is true that a vision of a demographic pyramid top-heavy with greedy geezers crushing the fiscal lifeblood out of a tiny cohort of people in the workforce as they indulge their insatiable appetites for ocean cruises, feeding tubes, and bright green golf pants is providing full employment for a whole gaggle of handwringers—the intergenerational warfare experts. What will become of America they cry as Social Security goes bankrupt, Medicare bellies up, and oldsters continue to demand the pensions and retirement benefits they were promised by the generation ahead of them who will be far too dead to care when the bill comes due? And dare oldsters expect youngsters to sacrifice their own self-interest and that of their children to maintain a giant gaggle of grannies and grandpas in affluence?

The problem of an aging society is ethical not economic. We need to realize that living longer is a good thing. We must also acknowledge that the elderly, just by dint of being old, deserve a dignified and comfortable old age. Once these points are conceded, America will find a way to make sure that the money is there to do what is good and what is right. If we do not acknowledge that living longer is a good thing and that old age generates obligations of respect, care, and concern, we will make the predictions of the intergenerational warfare experts self-fulfilling.

Prevention in New Jersey

New Jersey is not the first place that comes to mind in thinking about trendsetting for the rest of the nation. But the state comedians love to pillory is beginning implementation of a law that is both bold and important. New Jersey is requiring companies selling health insurance in the state to provide coverage for preventive diagnostic tests like mammograms, eye exams for glaucoma, colon cancer screening, and Pap smears.

It is a notable and depressing feature of America's current health care system that it is obsessed with treatment. The overwhelming majority of the trillion dollars spent on health care goes toward efforts to repair, palliate, or ameliorate serious medical problems. Our private and public insurance coverage reflects this fact. Need a kidney transplant, eye surgery, or chemotherapy for cancer? The coverage is there. But, want an annual mammogram, eye exam, genetic testing, or hypertension monitoring? Forget it! If you want to prevent problems before they happen, all too often you must foot the bill.

Why do we spend billions for treatment but next to nothing for prevention? Could it be that we have become so confused by conflicting messages about the secrets of how to stay healthy that we are missing the point?

Week after week, month after month the media, medical journals, your aerobics instructor, and your mother-in-law erupt with news that the key to good health involves the avoidance of radon, eggs, meat, dairy products, secondhand smoke, emissions from power lines, stressful workplaces, refined sugar, and lint. These sources then add that in addition to avoiding bad things the simultaneous ingestion of large quantities of fiber or vitamins or selenium or mushrooms or calcium and such is an absolute must.

But those who work in the field of preventive medicine and public health, such as Dr. Donald Louria of the University of Medicine and Dentistry of New Jersey, who played a key role in pushing through the New Jersey law, know that the road to good health is not hard to find. Aside from picking your parents so as to make sure that they are healthy and long lived, some simple behavior will help you stay healthy. If you stop smoking, wear a seat belt in your car and a helmet on bikes and motorcycles, drink moderately, get enough sleep, avoid recreational drugs, watch your weight, and exercise moderately at least three times a week you have the answers. Doing these things does not insure that you will not be run over by a runaway bottled-water truck on your way to buy a package of bulgar wheat, but those who follow these lifestyles have the greatest chance of staying healthy.

Sadly, our health care system spends relatively little time encouraging, cajoling, or even flummoxing us into doing these simple things. Moreover, it is not even oriented toward making even a half-hearted effort to try since the economic rewards are in repairing problems not preventing them.

The New Jersey legislation was enacted with an eye toward increasing health and reducing medical costs by pushing the health care system to do more about health promotion and prevention. By requiring coverage of basic preventive testing at affordable prices the state is sending a message that the preservation of health is important.

Some of the insurance companies in the Garden State are less than thrilled to have yet another mandate forced upon them. And some businesses do not like the idea of extending benefits at a time when they are striving to lower their costs for premiums. But continuing with a system in which you have to be half-dead before your doctor can be paid does no one any good. The rest of the nation should follow New Jersey's lead and insist that "health" be a key part of health insurance.

Managed Care

- Larry Stanford
- Your Money and Your Life
- Merger Mania
- Tell It to the Corporate Giant
- Privacy Goes South
- OB Express
- Virtue Is the Best Medicine
- Buying Perks and Sticking You with the Bill

Larry Stanford

How many times have you heard from a physician, health insurance salesman, HMO executive, or government official that you live in the country with the "finest health care system in the world?" If you watch the wondrous parade of technology that flows across our television sets each evening, from gene therapy to PET scans to laser surgery, you could easily think that you do. You don't. Juanita Stanford can tell you that, for too many of those who need long-term care, the health care system is threadbare and falling apart.

Larry Stanford, Juanita's son, died on March 9, 1996. No one is quite sure why. When he died he was only ten days shy of his forty-first birthday. Larry Stanford was severely mentally retarded. He posed no threat to anybody. Yet "the finest health care system in the world" let Larry Stanford die isolated, emaciated, bound, and sedated. His death and what took place in his life just before he died, as reported by Vernon Loeb in the *Washington Post*, speaks volumes about all that is wrong with health care in this country.

Larry Stanford spent his final days bouncing around a number of nursing homes in Washington, D.C. He had lived at home with his mother and his sisters for 32 years. But his aging mother was no longer able to care for him. He wound up going to a nursing home called D.C. Village. D.C. Village might not be the best place for Larry Stanford or anyone else needing long-term care. The U.S. Justice Department sued the facility claiming that 37 residents had died there from preventable problems such as infections due to terrible bedsores. There is no good reason why a physically healthy person should get bedsores. There are plenty of bad ones.

Larry Stanford acquired a severe bedsore during the time he was at D.C. Village. He was transferred to Washington's Greater Southeast Community Hospital for a special skin graft necessary to safe his life. Shortly thereafter he was sent off to another nursing home, the Washington Nursing Facility. This place had no experience with severely mentally retarded patients. When, after a prolonged bureaucratic battle, he was finally transferred back to D.C. Village he had lost 33 pounds, acquired another miserable bedsore, and had spent most of his waking hours tied in restraints.

How does "the finest health care system in the world" explain the fate of Larry Stanford? It can't. Why was a retarded man allowed to develop bedsores so severe that they almost killed him? How could it be that he was allowed to starve? And why was he kept tied to his bed day after day? No one in the "finest health care system in the world" seems to know.

The fact is that Larry Stanford was a poor retarded man in a nation that has not a clue about what to do with poor people who need long-term care. Places like D.C. Village abound throughout the United States. Too often the severely retarded and the frail mentally ill who lack money are warehoused and neglected. And no one cares.

The stewards of the finest health care system in the world show little interest in the fate of folks like Larry Stanford. Poor, frail, mentally disabled people do not score high on our social priority interest group list. What is worse those who might be expected to fight for decent long-term care for every American—doctors, politicians, clergy, lawyers, and the media—seem either not to know about the problem or have simply lost interest in it. Too bad. As Larry Stanford's family knows, the finest health care system in the world can prove fatal if you are not able to afford it.

Your Money and Your Life

Is managed care dangerous to your health? Is it unethical to ask doctors and nurses and patients to live with the constraints that managed care imposes? You might very well think so given all the recent media attention directed toward this subject.

Images of physicians with gags over their mouths on the covers of national news magazines do not do much for the blood pressure of managed care administrators. TV and newspaper exposés in which parents complain they cannot get their plan to cover the cost of a registered nurse to come to their house to treat a child with a devastating chronic disease, or stories of people left flabbergasted at the drugstore when the pharmacist tells them that the pills that were covered last week by their plan are not today, leave many wondering what the managed care industry is doing to their health.

Part of the problem for the managed care industry is that it is making bundles of money. Salaries and compensation for executives and administrators are often staggeringly high. Profits and returns to investors are, ummm, robust. Watching people who have nothing to do with the direct delivery of health care wallow in money is certain to draw the ire of doctors and hospitals, who resent this hemorrhage of money from their pockets into those of businessfolk.

Put aside the bickering over money. Managed care is in itself neither bad nor immoral. It is simply a different way to pay for health care.

In the 1960s, 1970s, and 1980s, doctors and hospitals were paid a fee for each service they provided. Today, managed care plans pay a fixed amount of reimbursement annually for your care.

Why the switch? Greed. Under the old fee-for-service payment scheme physicians, hospitals, and well-insured patients made out like bandits. Despite years of warnings from business and government to get costs under control, they didn't. Enter managed care. We are now paying corporate executives and MBAs lots of money to do what doctors, hospitals, and well-insured patients would not—curb their appetites for more and more costly care.

Think of the managed care industry as a personal trainer and yourself as an unhappy bloated tub. The trainer's job is to get you skinny. The skinnier you get the more the trainer makes. In this situation would you feel safe not putting any limits or boundaries on what the trainer can do to get you in shape? I doubt it.

We need to debate and decide what boundaries ought to apply to managed care. I will humbly offer a few suggestions. Government should demand full public disclosure from all managed care plans in plain English about the nature of the care they give and the complaints that each plan accrues each year. Shouldn't managed care plans have at least some patients on their boards who can keep an eye on coverage and reimbursement decisions? State authorities and insurance departments should be able to perform audits on-demand to check on quality of care and costs. How about minimal consumer protection modeled after the regulation now used for the electric, water, gas, and phone companies where those with complaints can get a hearing? Any interest in setting limits on how much plans can earn or keep in their reserves?

Today you and I are at the mercy of a legion of businesspeople who you and I hired to curb our health care appetites. We need to be sure they do not get too enthusiastic about their work lest we wind up dead.

Merger Mania

Big, giant, enormous, colossal, and supercolossal. What do these words describe? Nope, sorry, olives is the wrong answer. The right answer is health care. Over the past few years some of the biggest corporations providing health care services got a whole lot bigger. The most recent to show a growth spurt is Aetna, Inc. the new offspring of U.S. Healthcare and Aetna Life and Casualty. Aetna, Inc. is now a $9 billion gargantuan that is the fourth largest HMO in the United States. This megacorporate marriage follows hard on the heels of Columbia-HCA Hospital Corporation's purchase of Blue Cross Blue Shield of Ohio and United Healthcare Corporation's billion dollar buyout of Metrahealth from Metropolitan Life and the Travelers Life Insurance companies.

This frenzy of merger mania certainly makes those holding stocks in the newly reconfigured companies happy. The corporate executives involved are pleased too as they watch their generous stock packages soar in value. Well so what? Isn't it just sour grapes to bellyache when somebody else makes a killing from running a successful business? There isn't anything intrinsically wrong if nine corporate behemoths now provide health care to one of every eight Americans. Or is there? Does humongous and profitable mean better?

Well, giants can drive harder some pretty tough bargains. Super-colossi have the will and the means to consolidate services, buy drugs, equipment, and supplies cheaply in bulk, negotiate lower prices from providers, and to keep computerized track of what is going on in the provision of care. Don't let those sappy TV ads and billboards touting lazy good times and languid summer afternoons that health care leviathons are so fond of fool you. In the world of corporate medicine, no one is sipping lemonade or lounging in a rocking chair when the bottom line is the bottom line.

Megahealth care conglomerates have reined in costs while making great money doing so. But can you feel secure even if you or your boss is paying less for health care?

If you are unhappy with your giganto health care provider, what will you do? Well, if there are only a few providers to buy from and if your boss buys your coverage for you, then you cannot simply move your coverage or care to another firm. And if you decide to take on one of the newly constituted megamedical outfits because of a gripe or a complaint, it will be you on one side and the representatives of a multibillion-dollar corporation on the other.

The downside of merger mania in health care is that the consumer may wind up with fewer choices and even far less accountability.

Decisions about coverage, what is available in the pharmacy, which specialists can be seen, or when to pay for new forms of treatment will be made in oak-paneled rooms by people who could care less and less about any particular patient's wants or values.

The only way to insure that the newly formed immensities that now dominate the health care landscape stay well behaved is to put some public oversight in place that insures patient accountability. As profit-oriented enormities increase their grip on your health care dollar, there is insufficient state and federal regulation to guarantee that business ethics does not become the only ethic of American health care.

Tell It to the Corporate Giant

Suppose your doctor told you that you needed a particular drug to treat your high blood pressure, headaches, or arthritis. Would it matter to you if the doctor owned the company that manufactured the drug? Sure it would. In order to rely on the advice you get from your doctor it is important that you know that, as far as the doctor is concerned, your best interest comes first. So why is it that the media and those in the health care professions have had so little to say about the enormous potential conflicts of interest that are beginning to surface in our health care system as those who make and manufacture drugs, devices, and other health care products begin buying hospitals, nursing homes, and HMOs?

Zeneca Pharmaceutical, a giant highly reputable British drug company with revenues of $6.5 billion worldwide, bought Salick Health Care, a Los Angeles-based health service chain. Salick provides kidney dialysis and cancer care nationwide to the tune of $150 million per year. Why might Zeneca want to own Salick? Salick operates ten cancer centers around the country at teaching and community hospitals. The company also owns and operates an HMO in the Miami area, nine dialysis clinics in California, and provides dialysis services in 21 hospitals scattered throughout the country.

Zeneca sells drugs that many of the doctors, nurses, and pharmacists working in the fields of cancer and kidney dialysis might use. The sale of cancer drugs accounted for 30 percent of the company's sales. Since billions of dollars are spent each year in the United States on drugs to battle cancer and kidney disease, it is not hard to imagine the executives at Zeneca drooling at the prospect of owning a company whose doctors prescribe drugs for loads of patients.

But the advantages to Zeneca of owning Salick do not stop with gaining control of what is in the medicine cabinet at dozens of cancer clinics and dialysis centers. Zeneca now has direct access to information on patients in the Salick system. This means the pharmaceutical company can monitor what other drugs patients are using. The prescription practices and levels of care provided by different doctors, clinics, and hospitals will now be subject to direct scrutiny by corporate officials at Zeneca.

173

When critics were eviscerating the Clinton health care reform plan they argued that there was no need for government intervention—the market would work effectively to contain costs and assure the quality of medical care you receive. When politicians in states such as Washington and Tennessee voted to scuttle state efforts at reform, they did so mouthing all manner of rhetoric about freedom from government bureaucracy and the right of Americans to choose their doctors. Baloney.

The greatest threat to choice and quality in medicine comes from a health care system that is moving rapidly toward the kind of integrated corporate monopolies that the old turn-of-the-century robber barons of oil, steel, and railroads could only dream about. Unless some oversight and public accountability is put into our health care system the only choices you and your doctor will make about the medications you can get and the treatments you receive will be made by business executives with MBAs who use calculators instead of stethoscopes to diagnose what is wrong with you.

Privacy Goes South

If there is one value Americans say they care about it is privacy. Throughout the 1996 political campaign, a parade of presidential aspirants and congressional wannabees mewed out paeans to privacy amid their other catchy and sincere remarks concerning their love of ethics, the need to always tell the truth, the importance of bridges to the future, and why their opponent hates little children, puppies, and grannies. None of these aspiring legislative titans seemed even dimly aware that privacy is dead. Nor was a single proposal offered about what to do about that fact. Privacy died because you and I have allowed ourselves to be bullied into killing it by the health care industry.

How? In the drive to contain health care costs, privacy has been thrown out the window. Your health insurance company, benefits plan manager, pharmacist, managed care organization, or state Medicaid program bureaucrat knows all about you. And they are adding to what they know every day.

I recently talked with Sharon, a woman who had just found out she needed treatment for a mental illness. She lives in a small town in southern New Jersey. She has her health care coverage through her company, a relatively small firm where she has been employed for 20 years. The employer has contracted with a managed care organization to provide benefits to workers like Sharon.

When a physician told Sharon that she needed treatment for depression, she immediately asked for a referral to someone who could help. Unlike some workers, her company's plan does cover mental health benefits. She was referred to a clinical psychologist for further tests and an interview.

The clinical psychologist agreed that she needed treatment. But before that could happen, he told her that she had to fill out a form in order to get the costs of therapy reimbursed. The form was an agreement to let the managed care company review her medical records but did not specify who would do that or who else would get the information about her depression. In a small firm Sharon was worried that something she wanted to keep confidential would be known by all if anyone in the company were to see her records.

What is worse, the form she got was six pages long and filled with personal questions about her sex life, personal relationships with family members, interactions with other people at the company, demands for information about criminal arrests, domestic violence, spending habits, and many other equally personal facts.

Sharon asked the psychologist if she really had to answer what she felt were irrelevant personal questions. He said unless she wanted to pay for treatment out of her pocket, she did. He also said he did not like handing out these forms, but he had no choice. If he fought the plan over the forms he could find himself cut out of the list of providers the company would reimburse.

Sharon is hardly alone in being asked to pay for her health care with her privacy. For every Sharon there is a Rachel who will not get a genetic test for familial breast cancer for fear her employer will find out and let her go, a Matthew who finds that his pharmacist has regularly been selling information about his prescriptions to mail order houses who then target him for over-the-counter drug sales, or a Peter whose benefits manager notices that he is getting prescriptions for drugs used in the treatment of AIDS, parkinsonism, or cancer and tells others in the firm that he is sick.

Americans love their privacy. But we are in love with a phantasm. Unless we demand that the elected giants of democracy in Washington do something to restore it the only people who will enjoy privacy will be those who can afford to pay for their own health care.

OB Express

Former Senators Bill Bradley of New Jersey and Nancy Kassebaum of Kansas introduced a remarkable bill in Congress. The title of their law was The Newborns' and Mothers' Health Protection Act of 1995. The bill could, perhaps, be more accurately described as the Save Moms and Their Babies from Naked Greed Act.

Before this nation rejected the efforts of the Clintons to reform the health care system, the average stay in a hospital for a woman who had just given birth was three days for a normal delivery and five days post-cesaerean section. Now that the job of cost containment has been abandoned by government and doctors and left to the whims of the free market and the graduates of business schools, women and newborns are being shown the hospital door very quickly. Some insurance companies and managed health care organizations refuse to pay the cost of a hospital stay that exceeds one day. Three days in a hospital is seen by some bean counters as plenty if you have had your child via cesaerean section.

A few babies have died either because doctors were pressured to boot moms out of their hospital beds before they were able to feed and take care of them. Other kids have suffered brain damage because infections and other conditions were missed due to the pressure to save money by making quick discharges a key element of obstetrical practice.

The Bradley/Kassebaum law mandates that insurance companies let doctors keep women in the hospital longer without penalty if they think it is medically necessary. The senators are not alone in their concern that mothers and newborns are among the easiest targets of a health care industry that is becoming more and more obsessed with making a buck. Maryland and New Jersey have enacted versions of the Bradley/Kassebaum law, and a number of other states are considering similar legislation.

The problem with such laws is that they do not address the core problem. The issue is not simply whether the effort to drive down costs is going to lead for-profit health care companies to make you, your wife, or daughter stagger out of the delivery room and recover from the trauma of birth in the hospital parking lot. The way to balance the interests and welfare of patients against the economic considerations that are now driving the organization and management of health care is not by passing federal or state laws that protect particular groups of patients or mandate particular forms of treatment. If your HMO or insurance company is told by the state or federal government that moms and kids must have the right to stay in the hospital for more than a day, their drive to save money will simply lead management to turn elsewhere. If moms and babies cannot be tossed out the door, then why not those recovering from heart surgery, those recovering from a stroke, or kids requiring kidney dialysis or ventilator care?

Disease-specific or patient-specific protections are not the way to go. Our health care system needs a more systematic way to protect patients against greed.

The decisions made by third-party payers about what to pay for and what to reimburse need to be more open to public scrutiny. Those who buy coverage and who must live within the limits companies set have the right to know from their health care providers exactly what those limits are and how to challenge them. We must figure out how to get those holding the purse strings to be accountable for setting limits to what your doctor can order. If not, we are going to need many more laws to protect us when it is an M.B.A. rather than an M.D. who decides how much medical care is enough.

Virtue Is the Best Medicine

Health policy has taken a sharp turn toward cost containment in the past few years. Efforts to use managed care, capitation, efficacy assessments, group purchasing, case management, and utilization review to contain costs have been underway for many years. While efforts at the federal and state level to regulate health care costs have sputtered, private, free market initiatives, often driven by considerations of profit, have not. It is becoming increasingly obvious, partly as a result of provider and patient concerns, that the primary moral challenge to those practicing in health care for the rest of this century and well into the next arises from efforts to contain medical costs and achieve greater efficiencies in the delivery of services.

The source of moral concern is complex. It is a function of the tension between the drive to contain cost and the perceived professional responsibility to act as a zealous advocate for commanding resources. It is a function of concerns about the compatibility of business ethics with health care ethics. And it arises from the view that medicine and other health care occupations are not businesses but professions.

The forces that drive the economics of medicine are changing. Where once patients and their families worried about whether services were being provided that were unnecessary, whether care was being provided in situations that were virtually hopeless, or that a patient might be kept in a facility for a longer stay than was really necessary, today other concerns are manifest. Overutilization is an issue but the fear of underutilization is fast becoming a much more important worry.

Physicians are taught early on in their medical careers that their primary moral responsibility is to their patient. Zealous advocacy is expected on the part of every physician in terms of securing resources for those in their care. Current public policy is now turning more and more to the physician as the person who must control access to financial and societal resources in the name of the hospital, corporation, health plan, or society. The same physician is often left morally ambivalent and conflicted about guarding the gate to protect economic resources while at the same time realizing a professional duty to advocate for the needs of patients who seek to utilize those resources for their own needs.

True, physicians have always had to make decisions about how best to allocate their time and resources, but the limiting circumstance was their ability to help as many patients as possible while preserving the quality of the care provided. When society asks doctors to discharge patients because a plan will only pay for so many days of care, these are constraints that appear less easy to square, morally, with the duty to be a zealous patient advocate.

Patients and their families are also facing new moral dilemmas. When the fiscal goal is to keep expenditures in check and the means to do so involves different forms of managed care and physician gatekeeping, then families begin to wonder who is looking out for their interests.

A crucial element in any therapeutic relationship is trust. Physician advocacy is important not just to command the requisite resources for patients who cannot do so on their own, but also to cement trust between doctor and patient. Trust is the basis for the honest and frank exchange of information and for the patient's willingness to believe that healing and recovery will result from the physicians' ministrations. If trust is weakened or evaporates because patients are no longer sure whether the person minding the gate of health care resources is looking out for their interest, then trust is imperiled.

One easy way to see why markets oriented to profit threaten trust is to look at recent events in professional sports. The fact that so many fans of baseball, football, and other professional sports are losing interest tells us something very important about what an obsession with making money can and is starting to do to health care.

The Browns, a professional football team, played for many decades in the city of Cleveland. But, starting in 1996 the team began playing in Baltimore under the name of the Ravens. This by the way is a wonderful acknowledgment that the humanities have not completely left public life since the tie between the Ravens and Baltimore is Edgar Allen Poe! Many people in the city of Cleveland were distraught about the move by the Browns. Large men carrying fake dog bones, a symbol of the team, wept before congressional hearings on the movement of the Browns from Cleveland. They felt their team was disloyal. How could the Browns ignore decades of tradition and fan support and simply jump at a more lucrative offer?

Some Browns fans, ironically, like some fans of the Baltimore

Colts, a team that, years earlier, snuck away in the middle of the night to take a better offer from a group in Indianapolis, told the legislators that they cannot put their trust in professional sports franchises that pick up and move whenever a better deal appears on the horizon. So they will no longer be fans of professional football. There are plenty of empty seats at professional baseball games to testify to the fact that the perception that greed is king has soured many, many fans on that sport.

Some respond that football at the professional level as well as baseball, hockey, tennis, and other sports, is a business and the teams that move are acting like businesses. But those who follow football or baseball or basketball do not follow them because they are businesses. No one was ever a fan of a business. They follow them for what they can offer in the way of virtues—both the teams and the players. Hard work, fidelity, loyalty, doggedness, accountability, availability, continuity, tradition—these are the traits that make people into fans. When money is seen to be the be-all and end-all of sports, then the virtues wither and fans begin to lose interest.

What does this have to do with health care? Plenty. The saga of embittered sports fans has quite a bit to do with health care and the moral crisis that seems omnipresent in rehabilitation and in other areas of health care as well.

Why are people in Cleveland, Houston, Minneapolis, Los Angeles, and many other cities upset about the relocations in football, hockey, and other professional sports? They are angry at market failure. In pro sports the market now says, if you have a team and someone else has the money, and wants your team to relocate, the team will move if the price is right. There is no such thing as loyalty, fidelity, a sense of community, tradition, or trust.

Those are all virtues. Virtues and values do not fare well in a bottom-line, profit-oriented market. The market in professional sports is distributing teams efficiently, but it is not giving fans what they want, teams that they can feel loyal to and players and owners they can trust. If a pure, bottom-line, maximize economic efficiency market does not work in sports team distribution, is there any reason to presume it will do a better job in preserving the virtues people even more fervently expect from their health care providers as money and profit become the sole guides to the distribution of health care resources?

Many of the virtues that patients expect in their doctors are not likely to be there in a purely economically oriented, free market system. Big corporations that lack local ties are more attentive to the fiscal concerns of their investors than they are to the specific local concerns of any facility or family. Just as it true with sports teams, owners can swap facilities, close them, or even literally move them as economics dictate. Administrators can order doctors and nurses and therapists to change the way they practice with attention only on the economic consequences of practice, not the moral compromise such emphases sometimes entail for the provider. And it is very hard to trust or exhibit loyalty toward a large corporation whose CEOs make hundreds of millions of dollars.

An unregulated market confronts patients with a system whose savings are great but whose virtues are few. If the patients being cared for are especially disabled, frail, and vulnerable, the absence of virtue will prove especially bothersome. Medicine, like professional sports, is very much in danger of losing some of its standing and societal status if trust is allowed to evaporate through the heat of the marketplace.

Today the economics of health care have shifted. And the private sector, the nonmedical private sector, is being asked to do the job of constraining health care costs. Now efficiency and profit margins loom in the calculus of what services are provided and who provides them. Patients must worry whether their care will suffer in the name of commercial interests and stockholder concerns. The only way to protect against the fate that has befallen professional sports is to place ethical values squarely at the center not just of physician conduct but of all health care.

It will not do for those in medicine merely to lament the loss of autonomy and control to businesspeople. Americans want costs constrained. But they do not want to lose trust in their doctors. And those in medicine must make the case that cost-containment efforts, be they for-profit managed care or other strategies, that compromise their ability to advocate zealously for those in the care, are immoral and unacceptable. They must make this case not only to their peers but to administrators, the media, the public, and legislators.

Further, there should be a political mechanism put in place to make sure that decisions about health care are public and accountable. There should not be any less accountability for health care for the disabled and the impaired than is in place for communications, nuclear and electric power, t.v. advertising, and food and water.

There is nothing intrinsically wrong with trying to make money from the provision of health care. But decisions about major resource constraint must be made in ways that are public, accountable, and the product of consensus. It is immoral to place the burden of gatekeeping on the provider at the bedside, especially the doctor, because to do so places in jeopardy the very virtues essential for trust and thus for good quality health care.

There are those who would argue that virtue is its own reward. That is not true in medicine. Virtue is a prerequisite for success in health care. A system of health care driven only by a lust for profit and a quick return on investment is not the best environment to nurture virtue. If virtue is allowed to become a casualty of the marketplace, then trust and ultimately efficacy will soon be in trouble as well.

Buying Perks and Sticking You with the Bill

Does Medicare need reform? Well, not if you think using millions of your tax dollars to pay health care companies for coffee mugs, umbrellas, golf tees emblazoned with corporate logos, liquor for meetings of executive bigwigs and earrings, cufflink sets, and other chachkes is reasonable.

For years the members of Congress have been telling us that the Medicare program is going broke. All sorts of proposals have been floated as to how to prevent what would be a human and a political disaster.

It is certainly true that sacrifice should be expected from every American in order to preserve a vital program like Medicare. But in looking for solutions to the Medicare crisis, the current Congress seems capable of locating only solutions that ask the elderly either to pay more or accept less. This is odd because as the Office of the Inspector General of the Department of Health and Human Services and auditors of the Health Care Financing Administration and the General Accounting Office report, the Medicare system is rife with corporate fraud and ripoffs. The Medicare billing practices of a large Georgia home health care company, ABC Home Health Services, Inc., which later changed its name to First American Health Care, raise the question of why Congress is only capable of demanding sacrifices from current and future Medicare beneficiaries as a way of restoring fiscal solvency to the program.

ABC allegedly submitted and got more than $14 million in illegal expenses for Medicare reimbursement. According to the *Biomedical Market Newsletter* the company asked you to pay $1.76 million overcharges in salaries, $1 million for conference expenses, and for corporate mugs, booze, golf tees, and earrings. Oh yeah, Medicare was not so insolvent that the company could not get it to shell out $84,341 for gourmet popcorn.

Several years ago, a major university was found to have included charges for liquor and flowers on federal research grants. Congress had a fit and began slashing millions of dollars in overhead rates from all federal university grants. Universities do not have the same lobbying clout as insurance companies, private businesses and huge managed care organizations.

For years a few corporations, some HMOs, and insurance companies have been driving up the cost of Medicare through all sorts of creative accounting practices. Yet, all Congress does is let hordes of lobbyists, many nattily attired in their Medicare-purchased cufflinks sporting their corporate logos, whisper in their ears about the need to point the finger of blame for the spiraling cost of Medicare at you. If you listen carefully to your congressional representative, it is clear that those inside the Beltway intend to stick those who get Medicare coverage with the solution to the program's financial woes. Before that happens you should insist that they also stick it to those who spend their days golfing, lunching, and wolfing down high priced snacks with your representative while putting the tab on your Medicare bill.

Starting and Stopping Care

- Angela Lakeberg
- Baby K
- Right Hand and Autonomy
- No Butts About It
- PSDA Stinks
- No Support
- Final Placement
- Back from a Coma
- Is Anyone Dead Around Here?

Angela Lakeberg

Russell Raphaely, the director of critical care at Philadelphia's Children's Hospital, stopped by to see one of his most famous patients at around dinnertime. The little red-headed girl had just cut her first tooth. He and the nurses on the floor were very familiar with the details of this young patient's life. She had been in the intensive care unit for 42 weeks. Dr. Raphaely was somewhat concerned because the little girl had had a bad night. The doctors had a hunch she might have a troubling lung infection. But he was not at all prepared for the phone call he received at his home only a few hours later. His patient had gone into respiratory failure. Her heart was slowing. Angela Lakeberg who, unbeknownst to her, had become a medical miracle and an American morality tale, died.

The cause of her death is still a mystery. Somehow inadequately oxygenated blood leaked from her heart into her lungs. Exactly why this medical catastrophe occurred may never be known. But it is not too soon to examine the moral legacy that Angela left behind.

Angela was born sharing a heart and a liver with her twin sister Amy on June 29, 1993. Shortly after birth the twins were seen by doctors at Loyola University Medical Center near Chicago. The doctors told the parents that the twins could not possibly survive together since the heart they shared was badly malformed and could not support them both. The Loyola surgeons told the parents that they would not try to separate the twins because of the poor condition of their heart and the complexity of the surgery required. When pressed, the doctors did say that other hospitals with more experience with congenital heart disease might be willing to attempt the surgery. The Loyola doctors told the Lakebergs that there was at most a one percent chance of one of the twins surviving.

The Lakebergs felt they had no choice—one percent was still a chance. They left their Indiana home and brought the twins to Philadelphia. By this time the national media had caught the scent of a gripping human drama: Siamese twins sharing a heart, flown to one of the nation's premier children's hospitals to buck incredible odds so that one might live.

However, the Lakeberg story took an ethical detour. The twins' dad, it turned out, had drug problems. He was using money sent by people moved by Angela's plight to feed his habit. He had a history of violent incidents and arguments. Perhaps, the media began to muse, this was a family not deserving of the miracles of medical science.

It is appalling to think that a father's vices are relevant in allocating care to a baby. Whatever criteria might be applied to decide how best to spend our limited health care resources, surely failure to fulfill one's required inspirational role on Oprah, Geraldo, or Sally Jesse ought not be among them.

The more vexing moral question raised by the decision to operate and the tragically unsuccessful attempt to save Angela Lakeberg's life concerns money. Was it right to commit more than $2 million of medical care, more than $600,000 of it public Medicaid money, to a long shot effort to save a single child's life?

Oddly, this should not have been a question for Angela's doctors and nurses. Their job was to do what they could for their patient, cost be damned.

Was it worth it is a question for the rest of us. Despite the fact that we are engaged in a national haggle over health care reform, the question of rationing, of setting priorities as to how public money ought to be spent, is one that has not crossed the lips of even the most loquacious of our elected officials.

Should Indiana Medicaid put more than a half a million dollars into a desperate effort to save a little girl at a time when thousands of kids do not get well-baby visits, prenatal care, basic physical examinations, immunizations, or even prompt treatment for injuries and serious illnesses because they lack insurance? It is hard to justify allowing the desperate need of one baby to hijack resources that could do more certain good for many others.

Angela Lakeberg should remind us that rationing care for children according to the sins of their parents is wrong. She also reminds us that it is difficult to say no when the need is great and the victim is a child. But if we are to get a handle on the costs of health care, we must learn to say no.

Baby K

Baby K was born via cesaerean section on October 13, 1992, at Fairfax Hospital in Virginia. She was born with a devastating birth defect, a neural tube disorder known as anencephaly. Two years later the United States Court of Appeals for the Fourth Circuit directed that the doctors at Fairfax must resuscitate her should she suffer a life-threatening respiratory arrest. This decision was so befuddled, so completely wrongheaded that it calls into question the ability of our society to utilize the cornucopia of technologies that have poured forth onto the floors of our intensive care units, hospitals, and academic medical centers.

Anencephaly is a fatal birth defect. It has two major presentations. In one, the skull is present but the entire cortex of the brain is not. In the other, the form that Baby K had, not only is the cortex absent but the skull and scalp are completely missing. Anencephaly in this form can be diagnosed without much technological assistance with absolute certainty. In both forms the only part of the brain that is present is the cerebellum. This is the part of the brain that controls basic reflexes, allows the heart to beat, the lungs to breathe, and the body to maintain control over its temperature and waste products.

Baby K was not brain-dead. Although she had some brain function, the limited function her brain was capable of performing ensured that she could not feel, see, think, hear, or in any way interact with her mother, her doctors and nurses, or any aspect of her environment.

Anencephaly has no cure. Experts in pediatric neurology know that eventually the brain functions that are present begin to wane and that, as a result, death is inevitable. While there are reports of children with anencephaly living a year or more, most children with the condition are either stillborn or die within a week or two after birth.

There was never any dispute about Baby K's diagnosis. Nor is there any disagreement about what that diagnosis means in terms of the capabilities and functions that children like Baby K possess. The only dispute is over whether the doctors who initially cared for Baby K had an obligation to do all they could to prolong her life if that is what her mother wanted.

As soon as she was born Baby K had severe respiratory difficulties. The doctors at Fairfax Hospital put her on a respirator. They did this in order to make absolutely certain they were correct about their diagnosis of her impairments. They also wanted to give her mother time to adjust to the tragic news about her daughter and to say good-bye to her baby.

The doctors told the mother that Baby K would die soon. The baby would encounter further severe problems in breathing. But the next time that happened the doctors did not intend to put her back on a respirator.

Baby K's mother did not agree with this treatment plan. She said that she wanted everything possible done to keep her baby alive. She said only God could decide when her baby ought to die.

For more than a month, the doctors and the mother fought about allowing Baby K to die. A consult with the ethics committee at the hospital was arranged and they agreed with the judgment of the physicians that life-saving treatment ought be stopped. On October 22, 1992, the ethics committee took the highly unusual step of urging the hospital to "attempt to resolve this [case] through our legal system."

The hospital did not follow this recommendation. Instead, Fairfax Hospital asked all the other hospitals in the area with pediatric intensive care units if they would take Baby K as a patient, but none would. Finally, the mother agreed to let her daughter be transferred to a nearby nursing home. However, she did so only on the condition that whenever Baby K's health deteriorated she was to be rushed back to Fairfax Hospital and resuscitated. She was transferred to the nursing home on November 30, 1992. Three times in 1993, between January and March, Baby K stopped breathing. Each time she was rushed to Fairfax where she was put on a ventilator.

The doctors at Fairfax Hospital thought this arrangement was bizarre. Why should they keep pulling Baby K back from the brink of death if the most they could do was to allow her heart to beat and her pupils to contract? After the three resuscitation episodes the hospital went to court for permission not to admit Baby K back to the hospital the next time she suffered a respiratory arrest.

The United States District Court for the Eastern District of Virginia on July 7, 1993, refused the hospital's request. The court held that a federal law, the Emergency Medical Treatment and Active Labor Act of 1992 (EMTLA), which prohibits hospitals from declining to admit patients in emergency situations, applied to Baby K. The court noted that Fairfax is a recipient of federal and state funds from both Medicare and Medicaid and as such is bound by all the requirements the government places on such institutional recipients, including EMTLA.

This decision was appealed. On February 10, 1994, the Fourth Circuit Court of Appeals, in a 2-1 decision, upheld the lower court's ruling. Baby K must be resuscitated whenever she begins to die because to do otherwise would be to discriminate against her under the terms of EMTLA, which is a law intended to prevent dumping by hospitals of poor or potentially expensive patients.

During the 16 months the courts pondered her fate, Baby K spent more than 120 days in intensive care. The cost of this part of her medical care is well over $200,000 paid primarily by Virginia's Medicaid program. During this same period of time the state of Virginia struggled to slash eligibility and benefits for its Medicaid recipients, including children and the disabled because of a state budget crisis.

There is a strong temptation to say that cost alone provides sufficient reason to stop treating kids like Baby K. But that is not so. Cost per se is not an argument for stopping the treatment of any patient. It is only when the costs of treatment are not justified by the benefits produced for the patient that cost is morally relevant to treatment.

Cost is relevant in the case of Baby K because Baby K cannot benefit from treatment. Perhaps her mother can benefit but she is not the patient. Nor is any other third party. Baby K's condition made medical treatment futile, impossible, and pointless and thus whatever cost is involved would be difficult to justify on moral grounds.

The moral basis for allowing children like Baby K to die is that doctors cannot do anything to fix or repair their fatal illness. The patient cannot benefit from anything doctors can do. The goal of medicine in cases such as Baby K is not to maintain organic functioning in the dying or to honor the requests of relatives to continue care regardless of prognosis. Baby K is a patient beyond the reach of modern medicine. As such the only moral course available to medicine is to permit her to die without forcing her to undergo an utterly useless course of technological interventions.

The judges who voted to require the doctors to provide treatment to a patient who cannot possibly benefit from it said that they saw their job simply as making the hospital adhere to the letter of the law enacted by Congress. Congress did not say that stabilizing, emergency care did not have to be given to babies lacking most of their brain, who have no mental functions and who cannot possibly be aware of anything in the world around them. By not explicitly exempting babies with anencephaly, the two federal courts that have looked at the Baby K case are saying that Congress must have meant never to let them die without trying to use all the technology and resources medicine can muster.

This reasoning is, quite simply, nuts. The members of Congress did not specifically exempt babies with no brains from the law they passed to prevent hospitals from dumping indigent patients. It seems safe to assume, however, that this is so either because members of Congress know nothing about anencephalic babies or they never envisioned any court being so rigid as to interpret their legislation as intended to mandate continuing rescue efforts for children born with most of their brains missing.

Nor did Congress have any reason to think that anencephaly would be included in the category of a disability. Even the Baby Doe statutes pushed through Congress by President Reagan and Surgeon General Koop in the 1980s made explicit exception for allowing the nontreatment of babies born permanently comatose such as anencephalics. There is no professional organization in the United States including the American Academy of Pediatrics, the American Academy of Neurology, the American Medical Association, and many other specialty organizations dealing with children which holds that anencephaly is a condition where treatment is anything but futile, pointless, and not appropriate.

The dissenting judge in the Appellate Court decision, Senior Circuit Judge James Sprouse, seems to have been the only person in the vicinity of the bench able to let common sense prevail over the mindless interpretation of arguably vague legislative language. In his dissent he notes that he does not believe "that Congress, in enacting the Emergency Medical Treatment Act, meant for the judiciary to superintend the sensitive decision-making process between family and physicians at the bedside of a helpless and terminally ill patient under the circumstances of this case."

Judge Sprouse is absolutely right. In trying to force hospitals not to deny emergency care to pregnant women and the poor, Congress could not possibly have intended to compel doctors such as those at Fairfax to continue to resuscitate time and again hopelessly ill, permanently comatose newborns. Even on a bad day, Congress would not try to compel doctors against their judgment and the judgment of the entire profession of medicine to use all of their technology in hopeless circumstances.

Baby K's mother said that only God should decide when her daughter will die. But she is wrong. Two judges of the Fourth Circuit Federal Court of Appeals decided when her daughter would die. The judges do not intend to play God, but they did something equally bad in the case of Baby K—they played doctor.

Baby K eventually died. But she lived far longer than she should have. Our society should take a lesson from this case and think harder about the need to define clear boundaries as to what patients can demand and what doctors must do when medicine can do nothing more than prolong dying.

Right Hand and Autonomy

America is a nation loony over individual liberty. Our obsession with individual rights and self-determination has really gone too far. If you want proof, consider the fate of the right hand of Thomas W. Passmore.

The 32-year-old Mr. Passmore was working at a construction site on an island off the North Carolina coast on April 27, 1994. Suddenly, he began to hallucinate. Passmore, who had a history of mental illness, thought he saw the numbers "666" on his right hand. Some believe these numbers are a sign of the devil. Passmore thought so too. Fearing that he was somehow possessed, he cut off his hand with a circular saw.

A short time after Passmore flipped out, a rescue helicopter arrived and carried him and his severed hand to Sentara Norfolk General Hospital in eastern Virginia. Once at the hospital events took an especially crazy turn.

According to various newspaper accounts, a surgeon told Mr. Passmore that his hand could be sewn back on. However, Passmore refused to consent to surgery. He said he would suffer eternal damnation if his cursed hand was put back on his arm.

The surgeon then asked a psychiatrist to examine Passmore. The need for expert input as to the mental competency of Thomas Passmore is hard to fathom given that he had just cut off his own hand, but such is the concern about not violating personal freedom in the average American hospital that this behavior was not seen as sufficient to disqualify him as a bearer of the right to make medical decisions. The psychiatrist, saw Passmore who diagnosed him as suffering from a number of mental disorders including manic-depression. She prescribed medication to calm him down. After taking the drugs, Passmore consented to the surgery to restore his hand.

Then, the compulsion our lawyers and ethicists have imbued in doctors and nurses to respect self-determination at all costs resulted in some truly peculiar events. As Passmore was being wheeled into surgery he started hallucinating again. He said he no longer wanted the surgery. The surgeons, more frightened of violating Passmore's freedom than they are of leaving him without a hand, wheeled him

197

back out of the operating room. Then they do what happens all too often in a medical system oriented exclusively to individual rights—they call their lawyer.

The hospital's lawyer punts. Instead of telling the doctors to get moving and sew the poor, disturbed man's hand back on, a consultation with a judge is recommended. Circuit Court Judge William F. Rutherford is told by telephone that Passmore is refusing surgery to have his hand reattached. The judge, who may not have known how mentally ill Passmore was, refused to order the surgery. Passmore does not get his hand sewn back on. Shortly thereafter he takes the ultimate step to insure that common sense and good judgment will never be permitted to trump personal liberty—he sues everyone in sight. His lawyer, Robert E. Brown of Norfolk, told the *Washington Post* that the doctors should have sought permission to perform the surgery from his next of kin if they thought Passmore was incompetent to decide for himself.

Well, I love my freedom as much as the next person but a nation that has created a health care system in which doctors, nurses, and administrators are not sure whether it is the moral thing to do to sew a mentally ill man's hand back on to his arm is a society gone over the edge regarding autonomy. If the price of putting some limit on personal choice is that a mentally ill man who injures himself winds up getting restorative surgery done even without anybody's consent then, nutty as it may sound, we might want to restrict our liberty just a bit.

No Butts About It

Bruce Robert Nelson's butt spent some time in a federal prison. The 41-year-old served a three-year term for possession with intent to distribute heroin. What makes his case interesting is the lengths to which the cops went to bust his butt. The cops got the goods on Nelson by having a doctor extract vital evidence from a location where the sun does not ever shine. How far can cops and doctors go to get the goods on bad guys?

Before his arrest Nelson was free to roam about the United States. One day he took a flight from Phoenix to Minneapolis. The police were there to welcome him to Minnesota. Acting on a tip that Nelson might be transporting drugs, Hennepin County sheriffs brought along a warrant to the airport that would allow them to search Nelson's "person" and possessions.

The officers searched Nelson's possessions and found nothing. This led them to take an interest in Nelson's person. A visual search of his body revealed nothing. But police work is not all glamour and glory. Out came the rubber gloves. Unmentionable parts of Nelson were probed. Still no drugs were found.

At this point, the cops brought Nelson to the Hennepin County Medical Center in Minneapolis. A doctor was called in to give Nelson's innards another examination. He felt something but was not sure what. The police asked that an x-ray be taken of Nelson's rear. Bingo! Medical technology revealed an unidentified stationary object where one ought not be.

The gendarmes asked Nelson what might have found its way into his nether regions. Nelson expressed skepticism that a foreign object had taken up location in his colon. When the cops went off in search of a laxative Nelson expressed something else. He carefully cleaned up what only moments earlier he had said did not exist and proceeded to swallow it.

The constabulary returned with an ample supply of aids to elimination. They strapped Nelson to a stretcher and forced him to swallow a large amount of liquid assistance. But to their surprise no evidence appeared. Puzzled, the cops and the doc again called upon medical technology to assist them. Lo and behold an x-ray revealed what had started at one end of Nelson was now at the other.

At this point the question of how far the police can use medicine to search gets especially problematic. The cops said Nelson had only two choices—surgery or having a special endoscopic tube inserted down his throat to retrieve the prize that the sheriffs were sure would send him to the pokey. Nelson, protesting, opted for the tube. After he signed a consent form, an endoscopy was performed. The procedure took about half an hour. Diligence was rewarded when the doctor fished a package containing 18 grams of heroin wrapped in cellophane and electrical tape out of Nelson's stomach.

There can no doubt that Nelson was carrying illegal drugs. There hardly seems to have been a part of his body was not used as a drug pouch. But the fact that Nelson showed imagination in the use of his bodily cavities does not mean that the police ought to be allowed to interpret a warrant as allowing them to force surgery or other invasive procedures to be performed on an unwilling person. Nor does it mean that doctors ought to go along with whatever the police prescribe for those in their custody.

In our zeal to win the war on drugs, worries about the likes of slimeballs like Nelson seem frivolous. But they are not. The police who order a surgical inspection of Nelson today might be arriving at your house tomorrow with a surgeon in tow to check out your most private parts if they suspect you of a crime. One way or another what Nelson managed to put in his body was going to have to come out. There is no reason to let the likes of him not only threaten the rest of us with drugs but also rob us of our right to refuse invasive medical procedures, even when prescribed by the police.

PSDA Stinks

There is nothing harder than declaring failure. But, sadly, living wills are a failure.

Never has an idea made more sense. The depressing spectacle of families such as the Quinlans, Brophys, Conroys, and Cruzans stuck with no options but to keep their terminally ill and comatose loved ones alive by means of medical technology because no one had ever asked if they would want to be kept alive horrified the nation. Sensible people of goodwill tried to find a way to avoid entrapping people with medical technology they would not want. The answer was the living will. By having people prepare written statements about their wishes and preferences before disease or disability left them unable to communicate, doctors and family members would have clear, indisputable evidence to use to guide them if a tragedy were to strike.

The notion of advance directives seemed so obviously sound that pressure mounted throughout the last decade for state legislatures to grant them legal standing. Nearly every state did. In 1990 Congress climbed on this fast-moving bandwagon by passing the Patient Self-Determination Act. This law recognized the importance of living wills and required doctors, hospitals, HMOs, and nursing homes to educate patients about them. The law also said that every patient must be given the opportunity to sign one.

Could any legal ducks ever be made to get in a straighter line? Living wills were obviously the answer. Easy, huh? Nope.

While organized medicine and the legal profession seem unable to admit it, living wills are a bust. A burst of recent studies and surveys pound home the dimension of the failure.

Well over three fourths of all Americans do not have living wills. Most people do not even know much about them. A General Accounting Office report on the impact of the Patient Self-Determination Act says that the impact of living wills on health care in America is "uncertain." This is bureaucrat speak for "zip, nothing, nowhere." People do not have living wills and as the GAO report notes even when they do it is not clear that anyone—doctors or family members—pays attention to them.

Why don't people have living wills? Doctors, the GAO report

notes, do not like to talk about dying and end-of-life care with their patients. One reason for their reluctance is that a lot of their patients do not want to talk about dying either. When the subject is dying, at least our own, most of us find other subjects more compelling.

Not only do people duck discussions of their own demise. A recent California study finds many, especially those who are Hispanic, Native American, or Asian, believe it is unethical to talk about their death. Many think it is arrogant to plan the manner of their deaths. Others think their families or religious leaders should decide their medical fates. Some think to talk of death is to court it. Self-determination is not something every American values.

Advance directives are ignored because they are often not available when doctors need to see them. The few people who have them keep them in safety deposit boxes, desk drawers, or in their lawyer's office. You do not need a grant to know that the last person your doctor will call should you die is your lawyer.

The best of intentions can produce dismal failures. While having a living will is certainly a good idea, living wills are not the answer to a humane death for the vast majority of Americans. It is time to head back to the drawing board to seek new approaches to death in a technological age.

No Support

There is no more dangerous place to die than an American hospital. We have made a complete hash of dying, turning it into a lonely, isolated, painful, and expensive process. Short of legalizing euthanasia, no one has a clue about what to do about this fact. If you doubt the sorry state of how we die take a look at the findings of what is known as the Support study published in the November 29, 1996 issue of the *Journal of the American Medical Association.*

The study looked at the treatment in five well-known hospitals of 4,301 adult patients who were not likely to live more than six months. They found that fewer than half of the physicians knew when their patients wanted no effort made at resuscitation or CPR. The average number of days spent in intensive care on a mechanical respirator or completely comatose before someone died was eight. Half of the family members interviewed felt that their loved one had experienced moderate or severe pain some time during their last three days of life.

Having discovered that too many terminally ill people are being too aggressively treated, with the inexcusable exception of pain control, for far too long, the Support investigators came up with an educational program to alleviate all this misery. Highly trained nurses were assigned to 2,652 patients who were just as sick as the group previously studied. These nurses talked directly with the patients and their families about pain control, preferences about resuscitation and CPR, advance directives, living wills, and their dire prognoses. On average they met with patients, families, and their physicians four times during the roughly six months before each patient died.

The result of these intensive educational and communication efforts—nothing. There was no difference whatsoever in the group of patients where nurse advocates diligently tried to inform patients and doctors about their options and solicit their views about dying as compared with a similar group of dying patients who were not assigned a special facilitator. There were just as many days spent in pain, hitched in a coma to a respirator while dying and just as many unwanted attempts at CPR.

The researchers conclude their ghastly report with the gingerly worded statement that "the study certainly casts a pall over any claim that if the health care system is given additional resources for collaborative decision making . . . improvements will occur." Well, not just a pall but a 500-ton dead weight. We die miserably and this study makes it clear we have not a clue what to do to fix the problem.

A start would be to admit that death is taking place in the wrong settings for the wrong reasons. Death is not simply a biological event to be managed by technology. It is an emotional event that involves both patient and family. It has as much to do with guilt, sin, regret, and redemption as it does CPR and respirators. In the intensive care unit there are far too many who are handy with a respirator but not much good at conversation, spiritual support, or the administration of painkillers. Until the terminally ill can die in settings where people have the time and the skills to permit a peaceful and humane death, too many of us will continue to spend huge sums of money to die in ways we do not want in places we would never wish to be.

Final Placement

Can the shock and stress associated with moving an elderly person from home to hospital or nursing home to hospital kill them? Lots of people think so. But it is not so.

I have asked a large number of health care professionals with significant experience in dealing with the elderly whether moving a patient can result in death. They all acknowlege that a patient could be hurt during a transfer. Injuries aside, every one of them rejected the claim that moving a patient from one setting to another, changing the environment in which they live and receive care, poses a lethal risk or can be implicated as a cause of a person's death.

So why do so many people believe that sending mom or sis to the nursing home is what killed them? Elderly and frail people die. Some die when they are moved from home to nursing home, home to ambulance, nursing home to hospital, or hospital to hospice because that is when death comes. They die, not because their setting is changed, but because they are old, frail, and suffering from a life-threatening disease. The law of large numbers means that some elderly patients with severe emphysema or weak hearts are going to die within the next week or two whether they go to the nursing home with a smile on their face and a sigh of relief at finally being able to be away from the kids or, spitting in the eye of the bastards who sent them to the hellhole that now must be called home.

So what is going on? Why are we so convinced we might kill mom or dad by making them go where they did not want to go?

Most people do not want to go to nursing homes. They hate them. They fear them. Every adult whom I have ever heard describe the decision to send a parent to a nursing home has done so with the firm conviction that, in doing so, they are conducting the secular equivalent of the ritual engaged in by some Inuit peoples of sending their frail elderly out to certain death on an ice floe. Health professionals who work in nursing homes or long-term care know all about these attitudes. Moreover, they know that the dread of nursing homes so endemic in our society is not entirely without a basis in reality. The conditions that prevail in all too many nursing homes are not conducive to safety, sanity, or satisfaction.

Why do people want to stay in their own homes? People want to stay home because they like familiar surroundings, familiar smells, familiar memories. They do not like going to live in other places for the same reason that almost no one likes to do without these familiar experiences.

Familiarity does not breed contempt when it comes to where we live. Familiarity breeds peace of mind since we feel safe and secure in environments that we have helped to shape and that reflect our emotional and psychological handiwork.

I hate staying in hotels. I can never figure out how to turn on the heat or the air-conditioning. I do not have this problem in my own house because I know where the controls are for the thermostat. I would not like the nursing home because not only could I not find the controls I might not be able to alter them if the building had central heat. Shifting persons who have established long histories with their environments to new environments may not literally kill them but it may so imperil their sense of the familiar that they feel a complete loss of control and autonomy.

Too many nursing homes permit too little individuality. They are sometimes institutions that keep too close an eye on their budgets, and the need to minimize legal liability. This is not so much a malicious or evil thing to do as it is a quintessentially bureaucratic thing to do. Nursing homes are not hospitable to individual patients but not because no one who works there cares. Rather, they are frightening because what makes places familiar to persons is that they have the opportunity to interact with and shape them so that they reflect a tiny bit of themselves. It is next to impossible to do this in the controlled and communally oriented environment of the nursing home.

Why don't hospitals engender the same dread images? Well, to be honest, for many people they do. But the fear of the hospital is lessened by the realization of those who face going there that they do not have to live there. Nursing homes are places people go to live; hospitals are places people go for a time in order to get better. Hospitals are never seen as homes but nursing homes almost always are. And homes should be familiar.

Sending Gramps to the home is to be dreaded because Gramps is headed to a place where the exile is irreversible, communication sporadic, the food bland, and the lights go off when the rules say they must. Gramps cannot shape the environment of the place where he is being sent to live, and he will not feel any tie of familiarity with his new surroundings.

The lack of familiarity is unlikely to kill anyone, especially if the person dwells in a location that has nurses and nurses aides available in a way that is not true in their homes. If Gramps has a respiratory arrest, he is more likely to get CPR and live in a nursing home than in his own house.

Those experienced in working in long-term care know that nursing homes are not hotbeds of individuality and personal choice. They also know very well that they are obligated to present all options for living environments to their competent clients and to their surrogate decision-makers if their clients' competency is impaired or variable. They understand that respect for the autonomy and the dignity of the client obligates them to maximize client options, explain the risks and benefits associated with each choice, and to work with clients and their families to make sure that coercion is absent and voluntariness undergirds all placement decisions.

However, case managers know that there is a big gap between the ideal of informed consent and the real world of options. If the goal of case management with respect to placement is to maximize the freedom enjoyed by clients by eliminating restrictions and obstacles to choice in the environment where the client will live, and maximizes the opportunities and range of options available to their clients, then informed consent can be something of a cruel hoax when the placement choices are restrictive and full of obstacles and the range of options is narrow. Nursing homes rarely enhance positive freedom; creating options, opportunities, and choices. They often are settings in which negative freedom; interference, intrusions, restraints, and restrictions, flourish.

Not only are case managers, (often in cahoots with families) sending their clients to institutions that are not and, as they are currently structured, cannot be concerned with the creation of familiarity and individuality, or positive freedom, but their clients must be sent there with their voluntary, informed consent. Yet, most clients cannot really exercise even a semblance of autonomy about where they will spend their final days since such decisions are often fraught with coercion and fiscal pressures. Offering options that may not exist to those who lack the means, the resources, the financial and psychological capacities to act upon them is cruel. Better to diminish the guilt engendered by a close inspection of the gap between what professional duty requires in the name of client consent and what reality offers in the way of constrained, limited, and tightly controlled communal environments by embracing the belief that clients should not be sent to nursing homes because their lives hang in the balance.

Patient choice, ideally, should determine placement for any competent patient. But the system that exists for long-term care is neither a system nor does it exist. The sole determinant for the case manager in thinking about placement for a competent client is what placement is most likely to maximize positive freedom for the client and to minimize encroachments upon negative freedom. When the client is not competent, the moral dilemma becomes trying to decide whether infringements on negative freedom that enhance the chance of positive freedom are acceptable and who is in the best position to make that judgment. Presuming families to be in the best position to make the call seems reasonable. Presuming the value of accepting restrictions on negative freedom, the right to be left alone, if balanced by corresponding increases in positive freedom, the right to do more and to have greater choice, seems reasonable as well. But neither rule seems reasonable if the only options available are not likely to permit the individuality and thus the familiarity that makes freedom worthwhile in one's home.

Are nursing home placements categorically bad? The answer is for most of them, yes. The litmus test is whether they are so constructed and organized so as to permit the individuality that would allow residents to feel at home in them, to find the nursing home or make the nursing home a familiar place. Most institutions fail this test.

The powerful, persistent myth of death by nursing home placement is more reflective of the recognition that we send people to a place where no one would reasonably want to go, then it is a realistic account of why elderly frail persons die when they are moved.

Back from a Coma

The headlines were everywhere. You could not miss them if you watched television, listened to the radio, or read a newspaper; "Hero police officer wakes up from seven years in a coma." Gary Dockery did in fact shock his family and his doctors by suddenly sitting up and speaking in a Chattanooga, Tennessee, hospital room.

Why isn't it an inexplicable miracle when someone wakes up from a coma? Those with loved ones in comas or who have made a decision to allow someone to die when a physician said they would never regain consciousness, need to know.

Dockery wound up in a coma as a result of a gunshot wound to his head. On September 7, 1988, Dockery, then a new policeman for the town of Walden just outside Chattanooga, answered a 911 call that came from the home of a man named Samuel Frank Downey. Downey was angry that the cops had been out to his house earlier in response to a noise complaint from a neighbor. When Dockery came to his house, Downey shot him in the head at point-blank range with a .22 caliber gun. Downey got a 37-year prison sentence. Officer Dockery spent the next seven and a half years in a coma.

Dockery was rushed to a hospital right after the shooting. He was stabilized but he required full life-support. A few months later he was transferred to a nursing home. Still months after that Dockery regained the ability to breathe on his own. For years he appeared unconscious but every once in awhile he blinked his eyes and would sometimes say short words in response to questions.

When he first went to a hospital Dockery's doctors rightly said he was in a coma. Coma means that a person is unconscious. It also means no one knows whether the person will ever regain consciousness.

Coma is often confused, as some hyperventilating media types did in reporting on Officer Dockery's recovery, with two other brain states—permanent vegetative state (PVS) and brain-dead. In a coma the brain remains active. The person may do very little, but tests show the brain is still active.

No one does anything who is brain dead. Brain death means exactly that—the whole brain has stopped functioning. Medical tests can determine brain death in adults with uncanny accuracy. Brain death is the same as being dead. For someone to recover from brain death would be beyond miraculous.

In PVS the brain still has some function but is severely and irreversibly damaged. People who are PVS may still breathe. They may even groan or twitch. But x-rays and other high-tech scans of their brains show such massive damage that, unlike for coma, there is zero hope of regaining consciousness. For someone to sit up and chat after being in a permanent vegetative state would be a miracle.

Coma is completely different from brain death or PVS. The brain is injured but it is not clear how badly. Charles Dockery fell into this category. His doctors suspected he would never regain consciousness. But they could not be sure. He did show some behavior that indicated his brain was neither dead nor irreversibly damaged. That is why they said he was in a coma. When he spoke after so many years, they were shocked, but the diagnosis was not wrong. Dockery died a few months later.

In matters of life and death, words count. Crucial decisions about when to stop treatment and when to try to resuscitate someone hinge on the difference between coma, permanent vegetative state, and brain death. Charles Dockery's case is an important reminder of how important those differences are and how critical it is to get them right.

Is Anyone Dead Around Here?

Why is it so hard to be dead in America? Brain death is the standard doctors use for determining death. However, it is a concept that many Americans do not understand or accept. The reason why is no mystery. Medicine and the media continue to make a hash of explaining brain death to the public.

Two newspaper stories are textbook examples of how to confuse and frighten people about death. One is a report in the *New York Times* about a horrible accident. The other, about a tragic case of child abuse, is from the Associated Press and appeared in the *Philadelphia Inquirer* and in many other newspapers around the country.

Twenty-eight year-old Leora Natelson was rollerblading on August 12, 1996 with a friend in New York's Central Park. She was struck by a speeding bicyclist and knocked to the ground. She struck her head hard against the pavement. She was not wearing a helmet.

After the accident Ms. Natelson was taken to New York's St. Luke's Hospital where she was put on life support. Shortly thereafter, physicians there pronounced her brain-dead. The *New York Times* story said that the doctors at the hospital then decided to wait for her family to arrive from California to get their input about continuing her medical care.

If brain death is really death, then why are doctors waiting to get input from the family about continuing care? Could anyone reading this story come away with any idea other then that brain death means you are kind of dead but not really dead? I doubt it.

The AP story achieves the same level of confusion. Malcolm Scoon, a 37-year-old doctor was indicted on August 14, 1996 for killing his five-month old daughter Mariah. She was admitted to Long Island Jewish Hospital in Queens, New York, on February 19, 1996 after Dr. Scoon said he found her in her crib gasping for air. Mariah Scoon was declared brain-dead by the doctors in Queens on February 21. The family insisted that life-support be continued. The story reported that John Cardinal O'Connor had stepped in to arrange a transfer of baby Mariah to St. Vincent's Hospital in Manhattan. She remained on life-support there until the story says "she died March 13." An autopsy showed child abuse had led to her death.

Did poor little Mariah Scoon really die twice—once in Queens when she was pronounced brain-dead and a second time almost a month later in Manhattan? If so, maybe a bigger headline would have been appropriate.

If brain death is the same as death, why are brain-dead people on life-support and why would a brain-dead baby be able to 'live'' another month? The answers have nothing to do with death and everything to do with human feelings.

In situations such as the Natelson tragedy, doctors want to allow a family a chance to see the body in a bed rather than in the morgue. Keeping a dead body in a hospital bed allows the family a more humane setting in which to say good-bye. In situations such as that of the Scoons, hospitals are sometimes bullied by someone involved in causing the death into keeping a baby on life-support because of their guilt over what they have done.

In medicine you can only die once. When you are brain-dead, when your brain has permanently ceased to function, you are dead. Respect for culture, law, and family feelings can lead doctors to treat some dead bodies differently from others. That may be sensible but the media and medicine must do a better job of explaining why lest people become convinced that death is just in the eye of the beholder.

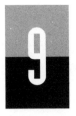

Assisted Suicide

- Kevorkian Loses It
- Jack the Wimp
- Loving Care?
- Euthanasia for Kids
- Waking from a Dream
- Australia Goes First
- Time to Die
- Death Takes a Holiday

Kevorkian Loses It

Judith Curren died at the age of 42. She was the mother of two children, ten and seven. Curren killed herself with a lethal brew of drugs under the watchful eye of Dr. Jack Kevorkian. Those who defend Kevorkian's euthanasia jihad as moral and humane had better take a long hard look at Curren's death. When Kevorkian did not see or chose to ignore a suicidal young woman's obvious emotional, personal, and mental problems, he firmly secured his rightful place in history as a dangerous nut.

Judith Curren suffered from a number of health problems. None of them were life-threatening. She had no terminal disease. None of her problems warranted anyone helping her to die.

Curren had complained bitterly for years of chronic fatigue. She had various immunological ailments. She also had complained of episodes of terrible muscle pain. She was using a wheelchair around the clock when she came to Michigan to see Kevorkian. The cause of her problems remains unknown. The medical examiner who examined the body after her suicide said there was no evidence of any medical disease.

Judith Curren had plenty of problems. They did not end with chronic fatigue and immune deficiency disorders.

Judith Curren was grossly overweight. She carried more than 260 pounds on a five-foot frame. She had a history of bouts with depression. And she was awash in domestic problems that had led her to bring two formal charges of assault against her 58-year-old husband. The second charge was made just three weeks before Kevorkian assessed her as a suitable candidate for assisted suicide.

What could Jack Kevorkian have been thinking when he decided that a 42-year-old mother of two young kids with no terminal illness and a long history of psychological illness, depression, morbid obesity, and domestic abuse needed to die? Apparently, Jack did not give the dispatching of Judith Curren all that much thought. Incredibly and inexcusably, he knew very little about Judith Curren when he helped her die.

Kevorkian had no inkling of the domestic problems that dogged Curren's marriage. When he learned about them only after Ms. Curren was dead, he asked, "How could we have known what was going on domestically 900 miles away?"

How could Kevorkian be expected to know what was going in this woman's life! Well, before someone helps end a life one might reasonably assume that you might want to know everything important there is to know about that life. When a 260-pound woman in a wheelchair presents herself to you begging for death because she says she has a host of psychological problems that are notoriously difficult to treat, might there not be some tiny obligation to see whether what she needs is better medical and mental health care rather than to be hitched up to a suicide machine?

There is no defense for what Jack Kevorkian did. When he aided in the suicide of a despondent, abused, and chronically disabled young mother, he completely blew his carefully constructed moral cover. Jack Kevorkian is willing to kill the despondent as well as the dying, the depressed as well as the doomed. His response to the frail and vulnerable is to hand them a gas mask or a concoction of lethal drugs. Think Jack Kevorkian is a hero? Ask Judith Curren's kids in a couple of years if they think so.

Jack the Wimp

Jack Kevorkian is a phony. Why so many people in this country insist on treating this flake as some sort of persecuted hero is impossible to comprehend. The death doctor revealed just how drab an object of support or sympathy he really is by his words and deeds during the circus that passed for his latest trial in a Michigan courtroom.

For years Kevorkian and his attorney, Geoffrey Fieger, told anyone within earshot that they could not wait for their day in court. Kevorkian would face an oppressive and unjust legal system unflinchingly with his head held high. Did not happen. Not even close.

What did the allegedly courageous moral pioneer do when the state of Michigan finally put him on trial? He stuck earplugs in his ears, a sandwich board over his shoulders, read a book while court was in session, and insulted the entire proceedings and everyone within earshot during trial breaks. His attorney pursued every possible loophole and gimmick to get him off. Kevorkian's courtroom strategy was evade, duck followed by weave, bob, obfuscate, divert, and waffle. His lawyer looked for technicalities as hard as any public defender might have in seeking to defend a corporate embezzler or a purse-snatcher.

In order to prove Kevorkian guilty of violating a now expired Michigan law banning assisted suicide, prosecutors had to prove that he intended to bring about the death of those he helped to die. The Michigan law had a clause which, quite reasonably, exempts doctors from prosecution in aiding in a suicide as long as their intent in giving high doses of drugs is only to relieve pain and suffering.

One would have thought the one thing that Dr. Kevorkian has stood for over the years is the duty of doctors to help those who request it to die. But when legal push finally came to shove, Kevorkian and his attorney showed no interest in taking a moral stand.

Attorney Fieger took precise aim at the "intent" loophole in the Michigan law and steered Kevorkian toward it. Dr. Kevorkian did not provide carbon monoxide and gas masks to people with the intent of causing their death. He argued that he had always merely intended to relieve suffering. Oh, please. What utter nonsense. Whatever else you may believe about physician-assisted suicide, lugging carbon monoxide and gas masks with you on house calls is not the road to pain relief.

Kevorkian says that the not-guilty verdict returned in this trial proves he has been right. Not so. When real moral pioneers such as Martin Luther King and Gandhi engaged in civil disobedience they had the courage to accept any punishment that might be forthcoming for breaking what they felt to be an unjust law. Kevorkian, if he really was a man of conviction, would have fired his lawyer, turned to the court and simply said that he had broken the law by helping four suffering individuals die at their own request. He did not. He waffled and used every technicality in the book in his defense to try and beat the rap. That lack of a moral conviction is precisely why his place in the right-to-die debate in America will appropriately be as the John Brown of the movement—a loony fanatic who stirred a nation to confront a very important issue but no one that anyone could ever take seriously as a moral hero.

Loving Care?

Nicholas Loving died on May 12, 1995 in Bloomfield Hills, Michigan. He died far from his Phoenix, Arizona, home because he had flown to Michigan so that Jack Kevorkian could help him die. Many, including members of Nicholas Loving's family, think that providing him with a plastic mask and enough carbon monoxide gas to kill himself was the right thing to do. But the fact that Nicholas Loving finally was able to end his terribly impaired life is no reason to view Kevorkian as a hero.

Loving, 27, was the youngest of the 46 people whose suicide Kevorkian has assisted. Despite his youth and the fact that he was not in imminent danger of dying, Loving's decision to end his life makes more sense than many of the other cases in which Kevorkian has been involved. Loving lost his will to live because a debilitating disease, ALS, robbed him of all control over his body. Facing the loss of all voluntary movement, he decided he wanted Kevorkian to aid him in ending his life.

Many, including Kevorkian and his combative attorney Geoffrey Fieger, have nothing but contempt for those who cannot appreciate the enlightened morality of what Kevorkian is doing. But they are wrong.

The problem with doctors assisting in suicide, even for a man as debilitated as Nicholas Loving, is simply that there is no need for them. America continues to believe that the only way to leave this planet is in the company of physicians. Either we must die in intensive care units attended by every manner of specialist and with a tube implanted anywhere one might conceivably go, or we must go under the watchful eye of a specialist in death like Dr. Kevorkian. This is nonsense.

No one needs a doctor, a hospital, or a piece of technology to die. All one need do, including Nicholas Loving, is stop eating and drinking. Death inevitably follows. Or a visit to the library or the Internet will produce instructions on ten other ways to die. Assisted suicide by physicians or other health care providers has everything to do with shifting responsibility, avoidance of guilt, and not wanting to be held accountable for what we do with our lives and very little with the need for help in dying.

What is worse for future Nicholas Lovings is that Kevorkian, by continuing his renegade euthanasia rampage, is convincing no one and scaring many. Oregon is the only state to move in the direction of making it easier to end one's own life. Voters enacted a referendum allowing doctors to prescribe lethal doses of medication to the terminally ill which they then would take themselves. They did everything in their power to avoid endorsing Kevorkian-style euthanasia. Whereas Kevorkian does not care about having special training in dealing with the terminally ill and depressed, mandatory waiting periods, second opinions, psychological exams, counseling, or even how well he knows his clients, Oregon insists that all of these factors be attended to before patients can acquire the means from a doctor to end their own lives.

Nicholas Loving and his family thought death was his only option. They have expressed no regrets about his death. It would be presumptuous to say they were wrong. Loving had the right to decide for himself when his life was no longer bearable. Even so, his suicide does nothing to refute the fact that legalizing assisted suicide by physicians is a bad prescription.

Euthanasia for Kids

The most momentous change in public policy with respect to health care during the past few years is the legalization of physician-assisted suicide in the state of Oregon. Those who favor this landmark change in the law insist that doctors can perform euthanasia without serious abuses. Oregon's law contains many protections to insure that no one is put to death without their consent. But a case from Holland, the country that has the most experience with physician-assisted suicide, raises the question of exactly how steep the slopes surrounding doctor-assisted suicide actually are.

In Holland, as long as a doctor reports an assisted suicide to the local prosecutor and it is clear that the person who was killed had made repeated requests for help in dying, was suffering, and was terminally ill, then no prosecution occurs. The Dutch Parliament formally adopted these protections into law. Thousands of people in Holland have asked for and received physician assistance in bringing about their deaths.

The Dutch seem to have avoided sliding down a slippery slope to involuntary euthanasia. However, their ability to stay off the slope is now in doubt due to a case involving the killing of a baby.

In late December of 1994, the Dutch Minister of Justice, Winnie Sorgdrager, announced that the government was bringing charges against Dr. Henk Prins. Prins, a 49-year-old gynecologist on the staff of the Waterland Hospital in Zandaam just north of Amsterdam, admitted killing a three-day-old baby girl at her parents' request in March of 1993.

The baby was born partially paralyzed with a severely deformed brain. Her parents felt that she was in pain. Prins killed the baby after consulting with a number of doctors who confirmed his prognosis that she probably had only weeks to live. Prins felt that even if the baby lived, she would not be able to walk, stand, control her bowel and bladder, and might have had a life of constant pain.

After killing the baby, Prins reported what he had done to the police and the local prosecutor. He felt that he should not be punished for what he had done since the parents had requested the death and since the child's life would, in his view, have been miserable.

Prins's role in the death of a baby shows how hard it is not to slide down the slope toward involuntary killing where active euthanasia by doctors is concerned. Once killing is allowed for those in the health professions, it is difficult to prevent the right to die from being extended to newborns, children, the retarded, the mentally ill, and the senile. The pressure to include those who are neither terminally ill—or mentally competent in the ranks of those endowed with the right to be helped to die becomes enormous. What is worse those who are vulnerable, such as babies or the retarded, to having others decide they ought be killed are much more at risk in America then they would be in Holland.

Unlike Americans, the Dutch have generous health insurance. Views about the quality of life in Holland are not as colored by the question of how high the meter has run at the hospital billing department. Nor are there public officials proposing to end all health care programs for babies who are the children of illegal aliens, new immigrants, or to throw all children of single parents into orphanages. The Prins case shows that the disabled are put at risk when competent adults are granted the right to physician-assisted suicide. Those who seek to extend the right to assisted suicide in the United States would be well advised to think harder about the much sharper angle of the slopes that exist on this side of the Atlantic.

Waking from a Dream

Ever been touched by an angel? Theresa de Vera, 21, may have been. That is as good an explanation as any other for why a woman written off by her doctors as doomed was admitted to Casa Colina rehabilitation center in Pomona, California.

Theresa wound up at death's door because the former Loyola Marymount University student suffered a severe asthma attack on April 20, 1996. Her lungs stopped working, leaving her brain without oxygen for many minutes. With no oxygen reaching her brain, Theresa became unconscious.

After the asthma attack, Theresa de Vera was rushed to Glendale Adventist Hospital. When she arrived she was put on life support so that a machine could breathe for her. But Theresa never regained consciousness.

She lay in a bed in an intensive care unit maintained by a respirator and artificial feedings. Her family and friends were always there praying that she would not die.

Six weeks after she had been rushed to the ER, physicians at Glendale Adventist began talking with her mother, Ruby, about shutting off her life support. According to a story in the *Los Angeles Times*, they told Ruby that Theresa's brain was in a vegetative state, and that she was not likely to recover the ability to think, sense, or feel. Her brother Randy remembers that on Memorial Day weekend the doctors began talking about the need for the family to consider giving permission to let her go and for "harvesting" her organs.

Ruby's mother did not want to hear about pulling the plug or organ donation. She waited. And she prayed even harder. The de Vera family are all very religious Catholics. They believed that somehow Theresa would come back to them. And, to the amazement and joy of everyone including her doctors and nurses, she did.

Ruby de Vera says her daughter's recovery was gradual. She began to grimace during tests or when blood was drawn. A few days later she called out her daughter's name and Theresa's head turned. Still later Theresa regained some ability to speak and move. The doctors and nurses were amazed. When she left the hospital several weeks later to go to Casa Colina, the head of Glendale Adventist could only say that she must have "been touched by an angel."

The de Vera family is very upset about what happened to Theresa. They feel that the doctors turned to talk of pulling the plug and organ donation before their prayers could work.

Theresa de Vera's recovery is difficult to explain. The doctors who treated her did the best they could given their experience and diagnostic test results to prepare the family for what was the most likely outcome of her coma. The physicians and nurses I know have a great respect for family values and for their prayers. But they can only practice medicine on the basis of what they know and what they have learned from similar cases.

Still, Theresa beat the odds. While she is not likely to ever regain all her health and cognitive skills, she has beaten some very long odds. And her amazing recovery leaves American law, policy, and morality with some real dilemmas.

America is stumbling down the road toward the legalization of physician-assisted suicide for those for whom physicians see no hope. When physician-assisted suicide becomes legal, what will happen to patients like Theresa de Vera? Will they be helped to die before they have had a chance to prove the doctors wrong?

America is racing down the road of cost containment in health care. Many now wonder how much saving money dictates what doctors say about the prognosis of those in their care. If families increasingly distrust what doctors have to say about the fate of patients like Theresa de Vera, what will happen to the huge number of other patients who, sadly, do not prove the doctors wrong? Will they be forced to live without getting a chance to prove the doctors are right?

Australia Goes First

Whimper or bang? Do important events in history start or end with a whimper or a bang? The bang theory seemed more plausible in the days of the cold war. Fears of nuclear annihilation were rampant and it was hard to imagine that anything important would start or end without a bang of huge proportions. These days, particularly in Washington, whimpering seems to be in vogue. Further evidence that events of great importance sometimes have modest origins can be found in a newly passed law allowing mercy killing by doctors.

A remote region in Australia is the first place in the world to make Jack Kevorkian's dream of doctor-assisted suicide on demand come true. With little fanfare and certainly no bangs, the Northern Territory Legislative Assembly passed a bill by a vote of 15–10 that allows doctors to prescribe or administer drugs to bring about the death of their patients. The Northern Territory is the first legislative body since Hitler's Germany and Stalin's Russia to allow doctors to engage in euthanasia.

The Rights of the Terminally Ill bill does carry some restrictions on what doctors can do. Written consent must be given by the person seeking to die and two doctors must agree to the request. A doctor with training in psychology must confirm that the person requesting death is competent. There are two cooling-off periods of five days and two days required before the doctor can kill the patient. If you are physically unable to sign the form required to request death, a friend with nothing to gain from your demise may sign for you. Oddly, there is no requirement that those who request death be residents of either the Northern Territory or Australia.

The Australian medical societies and church groups completely missed the boat on this legislation. No one in Australia or anywhere else in the world seems to have paid attention to the drafting and enactment of the bill. But what has started as a whimper in an obscure part of the world is now beginning to create a bang as critics of euthanasia in and outside of euthanasia realize what has happened.

Opposition to the bill is not confined to those who object on religious grounds. The Australian Medical Association is aghast. And aboriginal people who live in the Northern Territory, descendants of the original residents of Australia, are petrified of going to the hospital or clinic now that mercy killing has been made legal. They fear the new law will allow doctors to kill them.

Despite all the bells and whistles that accompany Dr. Kevorkian wherever he drives his VW euthanasiamobile in Michigan, it is a tiny Australian territory that has quietly gone first into the uncharted moral waters where doctors can kill on request. For those such as myself, who see no reason for involving doctors in suicide and who worry that allowing doctors legal authority to use their training and skills to kill will lead to abuses and mistakes, there is an important public policy lesson to be learned. Not all issues of ethical importance begin with a bang. Euthanasia arrived with a whimper.

Time to Die

A few months ago, while I was waiting to catch a plane back to Philadelphia I saw the Reverend Billy Graham talking on CNN. He was being honored at the White House as a great American.

Graham said he had been given a tour through the Congress, the Supreme Court, and other famous sites in Washington where he saw many statues and plaques honoring other great Americans. It struck him that these people had one thing in common—they were all dead. Despite their greatness, none of these people had known precisely when they would die. Graham said it would be better if Americans lived their lives aware of their mortality. Good advice.

But what if we knew the precise time our death would occur? As we move closer and closer to a society in which assisted suicide and planned suicide become morally and legally acceptable, many of us will. In all the rhetoric flying around the subject of the right to die very little attention has been paid to what trying to control death really means.

Knowing the time of your death imposes new duties. LSD guru Timothy Leary understands this. Leary, who died of cancer, announced plans to kill himself while logged on to the Internet via e-mail and a TV camera. Showmanship, pandering, and issues of good taste do not arise when death is an accident, but when your death is timed to the minute you need to worry about who will be there, what they will see, and what will happen afterward.

Presume the first signs and symptoms of Alzheimer's have now appeared and you do not think you want to wait around to see how bad things will get. You contact Kevorkian Enterprises Definitely Ltd. and arrange a dispatching on the last day of the month. Since you will be leaving in a few weeks, the folks at Kevorkian suggest, why not sign yourself up for a series of drug company studies of new medicines? The money could come in handy for your survivors. Or perhaps you would prefer to have yourself used to help medical and nursing students learn diagnostic tests and procedures. Discounts of 20 percent and more await those who get a little extra prodding from students prior to expiring. Or maybe you would like to select a mode of dying that will preserve your organs, blood, and tissues so that the usable material can be given or perhaps sold to others?

If haggling about making a few bucks prior to your planned demise is a little off-putting, how about letting yourself be experimented upon after your planned death for a period of time? Your corpse, maintained on machines, could be of great value to medical research. Why, it might even be possible to knock half the price off of an assisted suicide if you'd be willing to postpone your funeral for a few days.

Death awaits us all. Many believe it will be an easier meeting if they can set the date, time, and place. But the price of taking control over when you die has costs that we have hardly begun to understand.

Death Takes a Holiday

Death needs a vacation. He is getting a migraine. Dying is getting so squirrelly that it almost makes you feel sorry for the Reapmeister. No wonder he is grim. Consider the conflicting messages this nation has sent his way.

On March 2, 1996, Cardinal John Krol, a monumental figure in the Catholic Church, died with dignity. After months of letting doctors battle his failing body, the cardinal left Thomas Jefferson University Medical Center and went home. The 85-year-old former Archbishop of Philadelphia died peacefully with no extraordinary medical measures used to prolong his life. One of those present as he died was his close friend, Cardinal John O'Connor, the Archbishop of New York.

While Cardinal Krol presented a riveting lesson about how to die, it is not one that Cardinal O'Connor accepted. As Krol lay dying, Cardinal O'Connor was making arrangements for the admission of a brain-dead infant, Mariah Scoon, to a New York hospital.

Physicians at Long Island Jewish Medical Center had pronounced the baby dead after her father brought her to the hospital saying she had stopped breathing. The child's parents said as fundamentalist Christians they could not accept her death. Talk of possible child abuse swirled ominously in the background. The longer the baby was kept on technology the more difficult it would be to prove how she died. The parents went to court to compel the doctors at Long Island Jewish to continue using medical technology. It was then that the cardinal intervened and the baby was transferred to another hospital. Mariah Scoon's lifeless body was attached to the very machines that Cardinal Krol had foregone. No wonder the Reaper is confused. Even stranger messages emanated from the state of Michigan.

A jury in Pontiac, Michigan, refused to convict Jack Kevorkian of assisted suicide despite the fact that he had a canister of carbon monoxide with him when he paid visits to those who had asked to see him. As the innocent verdict was being read, 69-year-old Gerald Klooster was being held in safekeeping by his physician son. The son had learned his mother was planning to bring the Alzheimer-impaired Klooster to see none other than—Dr. Kevorkian. Family members immediately set about fighting in court, a battle that produced two completely inconsistent guardianship rulings from judges in two states.

But wait, there's more. A jury in Flint, Michigan, awarded $16.5 million to a severely brain-damaged woman, Brenda Young, and her family for keeping her alive. The family sued Genesys Health System for keeping Brenda on a respirator, kidney dialysis, and artificial feeding. Her mother told the jury she would never have given consent to these treatments if she had understood what they were and that they would keep her daughter alive in a severely impaired state.

While the courts and juries of Michigan were either urging assisted suicide, hiding potential clients from Kevorkian, or giving awards for violating patient rights by keeping them alive, an equally odd case emerged in Pennsylvania. Marlene and Tyrone Rideout of York, Pa. pressed forward in their suit against the Hershey Medical Center. They allege that the doctors there stopped treating their comatose baby without their consent, causing her to die. The hospital says that the doctors stopped treatment because further care would have been futile.

You think you got it tough. Pity poor Death. Sometimes religious leaders think going home is the thing to do. Sometimes they believe treating the dead with high technology is obligatory. In Michigan doctors can lose a suit for keeping patients alive but be found not guilty for helping to kill them. Some doctors think they must keep treating even when death has come. Others are brought to court when they stop treating when they think they can do nothing more to prevent death. Still others wind up on trial for prolonging life when the family does not want the patient to live. Yo, Reaper! What say you take a little holiday so America's doctors, judges, lawyers, legislators, pundits, and politicians can figure out what they really want from you.

Aids and Other Plagues

The Future of AIDS

Can someone with AIDS learn to live with it? Such a question would have seemed crazy only a year ago. Now, recent breakthroughs using a second generation of drugs and vaccines make this a legitimate question. Particularly since transforming AIDS from a fatal disease to a chronic one has important ethical and policy consequences.

For the first time in the history of the AIDS epidemic there is a sense of optimism and hope among many in the medical research community. Researchers are reporting some initial success in checking the rate at which the virus that causes AIDS multiplies and damages human cells and tissues. In one study at New York University, physicians got HIV levels in a few subjects down to almost nothing.

The drugs used in the NYU study had to be taken in huge doses, 15 pills a day, in a highly proscribed regimen. And the drugs and follow-up monitoring tests are expensive, in the range of $20,000 a year per patient.

These early tests are not cures for AIDS. Killing off lots of HIV virus leaves a person open to other sorts of infections and medical problems. And the AIDS virus has proven itself to be frustratingly nimble at developing resistance to even the most powerful viral killing drugs. Still, these tests and others have some scientists talking with newfound enthusiasm about finding treatments that will change AIDS from a death sentence to a life sentence.

Finding drugs that can extend lives is a wonderful thing. It is important, however, to take a hard look at what such a transformation in the world of AIDS ought to mean for public health policy.

Turning AIDS into a chronic illness is no reason to pull back on efforts to persuade people to avoid behavior that puts them at risk of infection. Persons with AIDS who live longer still need to be diligent about not infecting others and not engaging in behavior that would introduce new strains of HIV into their bodies.

And finding new drugs that can extend life carries with it responsibilities. New treatments will be expensive and even demanding. They will require a real commitment on the part of those who need treatment to stick with their doctors' advice. If the public sees lots of cases of people failing to follow through on their medications or putting themselves and others at risk, the political will to pay for the best available drugs and push on to find even better ones may wane.

And, most important, if HIV and AIDS become chronic illnesses, new public policies with respect to testing and screening are in order. In a world in which AIDS is a death sentence, when one's job and insurance can disappear overnight, should a diagnosis become public, when public fear and loathing lead to stigma and even physical attack, concerns about routine and mandatory testing and screening are understandable. But if AIDS becomes a chronic condition that is amenable to treatment, the need to start treatment early and to make sure that those who are infected get treated weakens the case against routine, mandatory testing. If medicine learns how to kill the HIV virus, politicians, civil rights activities, and AIDS activist groups must be ready to extend testing and screening quickly so as to afford the maximum amount of treatment to the greatest number of people.

Treatment for AIDS seems to be on the horizon. It is not too early to start thinking about changes in public policy that will allow those who need treatment the best chance of benefiting when it arrives.

Who's AIDS?

The United Nation's World Health Organization (WHO) announced that it is planning to carry out tests of two vaccines that might afford some protection against becoming infected with the virus that causes AIDS. The need for a vaccine is especially pressing since in many of the poorest nations of the world the AIDS epidemic is exploding. Yet, many believe testing vaccines in poor nations is unethical. They are wrong.

Many of us still think of AIDS as somehow peculiarly an American disease. Nothing could be further from the truth.

Just over 22 million people had become HIV positive by the end of 1994. Of those fewer than 5 percent live in North America. The rate at which HIV is spreading in the United States, according to a report from the Centers for Disease Control, is declining. The same is not true in many, many other countries.

Nearly three-quarters of all HIV infections, 15.5 million, have occurred in sub-Saharan Africa. In Uganda half of all deaths are due to AIDS. Another three million persons are HIV positive in Southeast Asia. The infection rate has gone up by a factor of ten in Thailand since 1990. The expected rates of increase for the next two years in Africa, Latin America, the Caribbean, Southeast Asia, and Western Europe are higher then those expected for the United States and Canada.

These depressing numbers are of great ethical and scientific relevance in deciding whether and where to test vaccines. The fastest way to see if a vaccine provides any sort of protection is to study a population where the infection rate is growing quickly. A population with a high risk of AIDS will require fewer persons to be tested in order to show a preventive effect from a vaccine. That is one reason why the WHO is interested in Thailand, Uganda, and Brazil as possible locations for vaccine trials.

The ethical problems with conducting trials of new vaccines in poor nations are many and they are especially thorny. In some nations rates of literacy are so low that it is doubtful whether all prospective participants will fully understand the nature of a test. Offering an AIDS vaccine may give a sense of false protection to those in the study.

Some third-world countries have almost no medical capacity for treating AIDS, making involvement in a vaccine test not so much a matter of voluntary choice as an irresistible opportunity. And undertaking a study of a vaccine in poor nations that ultimately will be sold at prices that put it beyond the reach of any except those in the richest group raises obvious questions about exploitation and equity.

Still, if it is possible to identify particular groups in poor nations who face extraordinary risks of contracting the disease and, if nothing can be done to reduce those risks, then doesn't it make sense to try a vaccine, even a risky, only partially protective one, on those who stand to gain the most from it? It does, but only if a few key conditions are met.

First, those who get the vaccine must face extraordinary risks of getting the disease—say sex workers in Thailand or IV drug users in Brazil. Second, every effort must be made to get those at high risk to stop doing whatever it is that puts them at high risk, even if it threatens the speed with which vaccines can be tested. Third, every effort should be made to obtain informed consent, especially since some subjects may mistakenly presume that if they have been vaccinated they cannot acquire HIV or transmit it. And last, those in the study should know that if the vaccine works it will be made available by the vaccine manufacturer at affordable prices in the nation where the study is done.

The ethics of conducting research in the midst of a raging plague are not the same as those that ought to prevail under other circumstances. With the appropriate safeguards, vaccine research in poor nations can be an act of compassion not exploitation.

Mandatory Testing

AIDS is the fifth leading cause of death among children younger than 15 in the United States. At least 4,700 children have contracted AIDS at birth from their mothers. More than 6,000 women who are infected with HIV will give birth this year. A quarter of their babies will be born HIV-infected.

These grim statistics might make one assume that if a treatment were available which could help prevent newborns from becoming infected with HIV, everything possible would be done to make sure they got it. That assumption would be wrong. A strange combination of politics and fuzzy moral thinking is allowing infants to continue to contract HIV when this could have been prevented.

Studies done at a number of sites in the United States and France have found that if women take the drug AZT during pregnancy, they can cut the rate of infection to their babies by two-thirds. Only 8 percent of infants whose mothers took AZT late in their pregnancies were infected as opposed to a 25 percent infection rate for moms who did not. In fact, the results were so impressive that the scientists felt that they had to stop the study prematurely and give AZT to all of the women signed up in the study.

These results would seem to indicate that every woman who is pregnant should have to take an HIV test. However, the idea of mandatory HIV testing terrifies many groups who ought to know better. Numerous public health officials, academics, and AIDS activists continue to argue for voluntary testing despite the growing evidence that AZT given during pregnancy can prevent babies from getting AIDS.

Some oppose any type of mandatory testing on the grounds that those with HIV quickly become the victims of discrimination and stigma. Others oppose the mandatory testing of pregnant women because they do not believe the government should have the authority to compel a woman to yield her privacy for the sake of an as yet unborn child. These arguments are remarkably unpersuasive.

Of course persons with HIV should not be made to suffer discrimination or loss of privacy. But when the opportunity exists to prevent the spread of a disease that is fatal, miserable, and costly, the answer is not to shy away from required testing but to enforce laws preventing discrimination against those with HIV. True, mandatory testing comes at the cost of some loss of privacy during pregnancy. But mandatory HIV testing with severe penalties for violations of confidentiality and privacy will protect a mother's civil rights and the health of her baby.

A pregnant woman who intends to give birth has certain ethical obligations toward that child. One of those obligations is to make sure that the baby is born free from fatal diseases. Society has certain obligations to protect the health of those kids who it knows are going to come into this world. If, by testing pregnant moms, it is possible to give them a drug that poses no risk to them but can save their baby a great deal of suffering and, eventually, death, then the right to avoid testing must yield to the best of interest of the baby. Babies cannot protect themselves against AIDS. It is up to the rest of us to see that we have public policies in place that do.

C'mon CDC, Get It Right

The United States Public Health Service has issued recommendations governing the counseling and testing of pregnant women for the AIDS virus. The guidelines urge that all pregnant women be offered an HIV test. Martha Rogers, an AIDS public health specialist at the Centers for Disease Control in Atlanta, said that the guidelines are intended to make AIDS education, testing, and counseling an important part of prenatal and obstetric care. But the guidelines do not go far enough. They recommend that HIV testing for pregnant women remain voluntary. It should be mandatory.

There are three very compelling reasons for mandatory testing. A number of studies show that the drug AZT, if taken early during a pregnancy, can cut by two-thirds the number of babies born infected with HIV. Quick treatment with AZT right after birth may prevent transmission. And, breast-feeding by a mom who does not realize that she is HIV positive is another route by which a child can contract the AIDS virus.

Last year about 7,000 HIV-infected women gave birth in the United States. Transmission rates to their babies are estimated by the Public Health Service to be between 15 and 30 percent. So, somewhere between 1,000 and 2,000 babies got the HIV virus from their mothers. AIDS is now the seventh leading killer of young children. Nearly 90 percent of these cases and virtually all new HIV cases in kids are the result of transmission during pregnancy. The numbers of infected women and children are growing.

So why don't the regulations call for mandatory testing? Maybe the answer is that it would cost too much to test all pregnant women.

There are about four million women who give birth in the United States each year. Testing all of them for HIV would cost roughly $100 million. But the cost of caring for a baby born with HIV is, conservatively, $35,000 per year. The children live, on average, about ten years. Each child born with HIV represents $350,000 in health care costs. Preventing 1,000 cases of transmission each year through the early administration of AZT or by shifting from breast to formula feeding will save $350 million. So it makes sense to spend the money mandatory testing would require.

It could be argued that there is no point in testing all four million pregnant American women since only a tiny percentage will be HIV positive. But the CDC's Rogers says that the reason for encouraging every woman to get a test is that every pregnant woman is at risk: "If you're pregnant, you have had sex. And if you have had sex, you're at risk."

Okay, if every pregnant women is at risk then why not make an HIV test a standard, routine, mandatory part of prenatal care? The feds believe it is because voluntary testing will get the job done.

Women who intend to have a baby do not want that baby to be born with a fatal disease. Given the facts about the benefits of early AZT administration, the overwhelming majority will surely choose to get an HIV test.

But why not simply mandate the test? The stigma and fear of AIDS is the only reason. Would some women avoid prenatal care if they knew an HIV test was mandatory? The way to minimize that risk is not by calling for voluntary testing. Make testing mandatory and it will become routine and mundane. If you are pregnant and are going to have a baby, your doctor should test you for AIDS. If anyone besides mom and her doctor get the results without mom's permission, then send the third party to jail. Moms who want healthy babies need information on HIV. Medicine and the government should make sure they get it. The antidote to fear and stigma and the way to be sure lives are saved is to mandate that every pregnant woman get HIV testing and counseling.

Sometimes Data Are Not Enough

Two important events in the battle against AIDS took place during 1997. One is the publication of a paper by a team of researchers led by Don Des Jarlais from New York's Beth Israel Medical Center. The article shows the efficacy of needle exchange, condom use, and other behavioral changes in lowering rates of HIV infection in men and women who are intravenous drug users. The article, which appeared in the *American Journal of Public Health*, adds more weight to an already impressive body of evidence that making sterile needles available to addicts so that they do not share or reuse them prevents the transmission of the AIDS virus.

The other major event was the decision by the director of the National Institutes of Health, Dr. Harold Varmus, to give the go-ahead to a $2.4 million federally funded study of the efficacy of needle exchange. The study is to be conducted among injection drug users in Anchorage, Alaska. The aim of the study is to find out whether it is effective to give away sterile needles to injection drug users and what method of distribution works best. The way the researchers will know is by monitoring the number of addicts who contract hepatitis B, a virus whose route of transmission is very similar to that of HIV.

The two events are not unrelated. The appearance of the Des Jarlais paper shows just how senseless and unethical it is for Dr. Varmus to allow public funds to be used to pay for the Anchorage study.

Ever since the Nuremberg trials at the end of World War II, those conducting research with human subjects have been obligated to secure their free, informed consent. A tragic legacy of experiments in this nation, beginning with radiation experiments carried out by the military on unsuspecting and sometimes incompetent persons, as well as the notorious Tuskegee syphilis study, in which the federal government allowed poor rural black men to be duped into believing they were receiving treatment for their disease, stands as a stark reminder that subjects must be told and made to understand all relevant facts about what is being done to them, why, the risks and benefits they will face in research, and what their alternatives to being a subject might be. Subsequent studies done at the Willowbrook Home on Staten Island, New York, and at the Brooklyn Jewish Chronic Disease

Hospital on subjects with severe impairments and disabilities established the moral principle that it is not acceptable to learn from the misery or ill fortunate of the vulnerable and the frail without at least trying to warn them and their guardians about the dangers they face. These core moral values and principles are very much in jeopardy should the Alaska needle-exchange study go forward.

The Alaska study is fundamentally unethical. It is using hepatitis B as a way to infer the efficacy of different types of needle exchange because the incidence of HIV in the Anchorage population of needle-using drug abusers is too low to measure accurately. But hepatitis B is itself a potentially disabling and sometimes fatal disease. It is also one that is potentially preventable through a relatively new vaccine. Knowingly allowing subjects to participate in a study without telling them that they may contract a deadly virus for which a vaccine is available is wrong.

The decision to study addicts at risk without telling them all their options and making at least a minimal effort to help them avoid death is bad enough. But there is more that is morally wrong with the Alaskan study.

The study is being undertaken in the face of powerful evidence, of which the Des Jarlais article is only the latest example, that making needles available to IV drug users saves lives and prevents the transmission of AIDS. Pubic health officials in numerous American cities and in nations around the world from Britain, to Australia, to Germany, to Thailand know that their best weapon against AIDS in the IV drug-using community is sterile needles. There is no excuse for not pursuing every avenue to get sterile needles into the hands of IV drug abusers.

Why then is the Alaskan study moving ahead? The answer is politics. Congress is leery of being seen as doing anything that might be construed as encouraging drug use. While the evidence favoring sterile needle exchange is there, the courage to do what might be seen as unpopular is not. Therefore, Congress has ordered more studies.

AIDS demands more from all of us. If steps can be taken to lower disease transmission and save lives, they ought to be taken. The point of AIDS research is to find out what can be done to reach these goals. When we know that something works the only ethical thing to do is insist that public health trump politics.

Inconsistent About HIV

AIDS is not like any other disease. How do I know? Try to make sense of the following reactions to what to do about the threat of getting infected by the virus. They make no sense to me.

A boxer, Tommy Morrison, finds out that he is HIV positive. Immediately there is a storm of reaction from other boxers, referees, trainers, promoters, sports writers, and fans demanding mandatory HIV testing of every professional prizefighter. The boxer himself agrees that mandatory testing in a sport where blood is omnipresent makes sense even if it means the loss of a career. Legislators demand action. State boxing commissions fall over one another to institute mandatory testing.

A young nurse, Lynda Marie Arnold, is infected with the AIDS virus when she is inadvertently cut by a needle while treating an infected patient. She immediately launches a campaign to insure that a safer form of needle, one that uses an automatic protective sleeve, is put into use. Only a tiny number of health workers have been infected through occupational accidents involving needles. The safer needle costs more than the standard needle, and because so many needles are used, the shift to the safer version will result in real costs to the health care system. But the many national AIDS organizations, health care worker's unions, and prominent health care professionals who support Lynda's campaign think cost should not be an object. Preventing even a small number of infections seems well worth it when it comes to AIDS.

Two studies appeared in the same issue of the *Journal of the American Medical Association.* One, a huge French study, involving 1386 children born at 62 hospitals all over France, reports that there are two forms of prenatally acquired HIV disease in children who get the virus from their infected mothers. In one especially vicious form of the disease, the babies are overwhelmed by the virus. They are bombarded with infections they cannot fight off, wither and die quickly, usually within months. The other form of pediatric AIDS more closely resembles the course of HIV infection in adults. The kids live for many years, some as long as ten, before the disease eventually wears them down and kills them. The course of the disease in infants, rapid and overwhelming, seems directly linked to the degree of infection suffered by the mother.

In the other study a group of pediatricians at UCLA report high success in preventing the transmission of HIV from mother to baby by using AZT during pregnancy and delivery. They state that AZT "exerts a major protective effect" in reducing transmission from women to their babies. This study confirms another, which showed a strong preventive effect associated with AZT use in pregnant women infected with HIV.

The reaction to these two studies? Nothing. Americans seem certain that the only reasonable course of action to the threat of HIV in boxing or among nurses and doctors working with needles is prevention regardless of cost. Not so for babies.

There has been no public outcry, no rallies, no editorial campaigns, no call-in-show frenzy for mandatory testing for HIV as a standard, mandatory, and free component of prenatal care. Despite the fact that the evidence is incontrovertible that AZT prevents transmission, that the earlier it is used in women who are bringing babies to term the greater the chance of prevention and, that the effects of the virus are far nastier the longer the pregnant mom has been infected, Americans seem unwilling to do what it would take in terms of testing and cost to reduce the numbers of kids with AIDS. Maybe if kids had a union or were allowed to box on TV they could get the powers that be in our society to do the right thing and make HIV testing a routine, mundane, free, and mandatory component of prenatal care for every woman who intends to have a baby.

Detention and TB

More than a year ago the American Lung Association convened a panel of experts to look at the question of whether state health departments should have the authority to detain, hold, and treat patients with tuberculosis who will not take their medicine. The final report of that group was published in the *American Journal of Respiratory and Critical Care Medicine*. Sixty-six experts in medicine and public health say government should give doctors the right to quarantine and treat people with TB even without their consent.

Treating competent adults without their permission is morally dubious in American medicine and law. After many heated arguments and contentious court battles, competent adults have secured the right to refuse medical care even if they will die as a result.

Too often we in this society tend to forget that individual rights have limits. When it comes to tuberculosis the limit on your right to go without treatment and die is when your decision puts the rest of the community at risk.

TB poses a serious threat to your health and mine. It is a highly contagious disease. Tuberculosis killed or sickened 11 million people worldwide in 1995. Any of those people might get on a boat or a plane and wind up in the United States. And some have. In a state such as Pennsylvania, immigrant communities experience TB rates that are 10 to 15 times greater than average. More than 22,000 cases of TB were reported in the United States last year. People with AIDS and other immune system diseases are especially at risk of infection from TB.

One of the ways TB can quickly move from being a small problem to a big one in this country is if people start taking medication for the disease but fail to take it properly. Treatment for TB usually involves taking four different drugs. Treatment can take as long as two years. If doses are skipped or people stop taking their pills before the prescribed period, the TB bacillus can evolve defenses against the drug and not only rebound in the infected person's body but also spread the newly resistant strain to others.

Every once in awhile doctors who treat infectious diseases such as TB encounter patients whom they think are not going to stay on their medications. These may be people who are mentally ill. They may be people who have failed to comply with medical advice for the treatment of other diseases.

It is the small number of people who pose the greatest risk of going off their medicine and infecting others with deadly strains of TB that led the experts to call on each state to give doctors the authority to hold TB patients who are likely to fail to comply with treatment.

Civil libertarians are likely to cry foul. The overriding principle of American law and medical ethics is to respect personal freedom and to allow autonomy to trump other concerns. When the only person affected by a choice is the one making it, respect for freedom makes sense. But when the person making decisions may not be able to do so, or worse, knowingly makes decisions that could cause the deaths of many others, then the right to be free or stupid or both evaporates. TB is too serious to permit a few to imperil the health of many. Let's hope that our elected officials get the message.

Lyme Disease

Do you think your tax money should go to support scientific research on the digestive system of ticks? No? Think again. Your life depends on it.

Congress finds it tempting to hack away at the budget for biomedical research. Support for academic medical centers is on the chopping block. Oddball areas of inquiry like bug digestion are prime targets for budget amputation. Too bad because, as Dr. Alan Steere of the New England Medical Center can tell you, the road to cures often winds along a very windy road.

I met Dr. Steere at a symposium at the University of Pennsylvania Medical School. You may never have heard of him but if you live in New York, Pennsylvania, Minnesota, Wisconsin, Massachusetts, or Connecticut, you may owe him your health. Dr. Steere, with the help of dozens of scientists, doctors, and public health officials all getting federal grants at academic medical centers and research institutions, identified and then found a cure for Lyme disease.

Twenty years ago parents in a few small Connecticut towns realized that lots of their kids had severely arthritic knees. The pediatricians in the area thought the children had juvenile rheumatoid arthritis, a very rare condition. The parents saw the disease exploding through their communities and began to press doctors and health officials to see if there was a reason for the epidemic.

The Centers for Disease Control asked Dr. Steere to look into the problem. He was a specialist in arthritis and also had been a member of a federally sponsored medical research unit that tracks outbreaks of rare diseases. Steere went to Lyme, Connecticut, to interview families and examine their children. He noted that arthritic symptoms first appeared at the end of the summer and the early fall. The kids with arthritis lived near big state parks and heavily wooded areas. Many had large red blotchy spots on their skin. He spent months putting together the evidence and thinking about what he found. He suspected the kids did not have rheumatoid arthritis. An insect-borne disease was likely, but what bug he did not know.

Steere showed pictures of some of the kids at a scientific meeting. A postdoctoral student in dermatology from Scandinavia working on a federal research grant took one look at the rashes and said they were tick bites just like ones he had observed at home. Steere went back to Lyme and soon thereafter found a tiny baby tick smack in the middle of a big red blotch on a kid's back.

Steere had the bad guy. But what did the tick give to the kids that gave them arthritis-like symptoms? He tried to dissect a tiny tick under a microscope but he lacked the skill and knowledge to do the job right. He needed someone who knew a lot about the digestive system of ticks. He found such a person at a federally sponsored research institute in Colorado. More months passed as many ticks gave their lives for science. Finally, a few years after he first went to Connecticut, Steere got his answer. The Connecticut ticks were carrying a spirochete (a kind of bacteria), in their gut that can grow in the joints of the human body. Transmitted through the bite of a tick, the bacteria cause the arthritis-like symptoms.

Steere headed to Yale and, armed with a federal research grant, began to look for a drug that could kill the tick-borne bacteria. A few years later he and his colleagues had one. Later still, work began, with the support of another federal grant, on a vaccine to prevent what we now call Lyme disease.

Chop federal support for biomedical research and there is no medical detective unit, no visiting dermatologist from Europe, no scientist specializing in ticks, no young rheumatologist to send to Lyme, and no drug or vaccine development. Devastate basic research at academic health centers that have made American medicine the envy of the world and all you have is a mysterious exploding plague of disabling arthritis ravaging kids without anyone having a clue as to what is going on. Before you let Congress vote to trim the 'fat' out of the federal budget by getting rid of grants for projects such as studying the eating habits of ticks, ask yourself what you think it is worth to have a cure for Lyme disease.

We Know Treatment Does Not Work

Every once in awhile science cannot make itself heard above the din of politics. That is the only plausible explanation for the resounding yawn of indifference that greeted the publication of an important study by the University of Chicago's National Opinion Research Center on the effectiveness of treatment programs for drug and alcohol abuse.

It is common knowledge that efforts to rehabilitate drug abusers fail. Anyone who has spent more then five minutes listening to Rush Limbaugh and the even dimmer bulbs he has spawned on the airwaves will know that drug treatment is a rip-off, a racket, and a plot by minority folks to evade responsibility for their addicted brethren.

You don't believe it? Consider the pathetic paths of public drug abusers such as hockey's Bob Probert, baseball's Steve Howe and Dwight Gooden, or basketball's Roy Tarpley. These guys have fallen off the treatment wagon so often that they wear knee and elbow pads.

We all know that treatment is just an opaque way of coddling addicts, drunks, and junkies. Enrolling those who cannot stop snorting coke, smoking crack, or shooting up heroin in ten-step programs, toney rehab facilities, AA-or government-sponsored drug abuse programs is just a trick to keep pointy-headed liberal weenies and their buddies employed. Better to arrest drug abusers, have the cops whack them around a little to teach them some respect for the law and, if they still go on using, insert them into the hoosegow for long stretches.

There is absolutely no reason to be concerned about the fact that thousands of women who are using drugs while pregnant cannot get into treatment programs. The programs don't work. That fact is obvious to anyone brave enough to stick his or her head out the window in any inner-city neighborhood in America to see the dealers, the drive-by shootings, and the eight-year-old kids with beepers. Except, as the Chicago study shows, what we all know is wrong. Drug treatment does work.

Urine Testing and Welfare

Looking to make some easy money? I got a sure thing for you. Dip into the nest egg, clean out the Christmas account, bust open the piggy bank—there is big money to be made in urine testing for drugs. State and county governments are pushing policies that guarantee it will not be long before you are urinating in a plastic cup two or three times a month to check on your drug and alcohol use. Trickle-down economics is taking on a whole new meaning and you can get in on the ground floor.

Congress is behind the good times soon to be enjoyed in the drug-testing business. It included a provision in the 1997 welfare reform legislation that permits states to test and then to bounce anyone found positive. States and counties are realizing that one way they can quickly trim their budgets is to get rid of welfare recipients.

Hordes of local bureaucrats and politicians are putting their imaginations to use trying to figure out how to make life especially miserable for the poor wretches who depend on handouts for their survival. While state and county officials evince little ability to link work and welfare in any meaningful way, prevent the vast laundering of money that is a necessity for the drug trade to flourish, or stop the flood of drugs into your city or town, they are mighty good at conjuring up ways to make sure that drunks and addicts are not living it up at your expense.

South Carolina is implementing a program for required urine testing on 45,000 welfare recipients. If state social service workers suspect drug use, they can require random urine testing. It is not clear what might trigger a state official's suspicions but given the desire to save money it will probably not take much.

If, during mandatory testing, someone is found to be positive, South Carolina Department of Social Services personnel say the recipient will be "sanctioned." In plain English, that means if you test positive your days of living it up on welfare are over.

People will soon be coerced into providing samples at the county level as well. A program for required drug testing has started in St. Johns County, Florida. *The Washington Post* reports that anyone applying for any social service in the county, including not only welfare but also health care and any other county service, must pee first.

The problem with all this government mandated excretion is that it is completely punitive. Local officials are not looking for ways to expand treatment programs, offer counseling, or put those who use drugs or booze into rehabilitation. The only reason to throw the civil rights of those who use drugs out the window is to save money.

Of course if saving money is the goal, why stop with welfare recipients? Why not mandatory drug testing for anyone who accepts an agricultural or tobacco subsidy? Or a student loan? Or any federal health care coverage? Shouldn't all federal, state, and county workers be asked to head to the bathroom each month and aim carefully before they accept their monthly taxpayer-supported paycheck. And for that matter, how about those federal and state legislators who are so eager to have others piddle on demand—shouldn't they get their bodily fluids examined to insure that they deserve the benefits and perks of office?

The demand for drug testing will only continue to grow. We have grown so weary of trying to find answers to poverty and drugs that we are willing to flush our civil liberties right down the drain.

Smoking and Other Bad Habits

What Was Bob Dole Smoking?

What was Bob Dole smoking? Certainly something that addled his mind. There is no other way to explain his bizarre statements on the subject of tobacco. No one would care what the defeated presidential candidate had to say about the dangers of smoking except that so many other Americans believe it too.

Bob Dole did not smoke but he did not seem to care very much if you do. Nor does Congress. They seem indifferent to the fact that cigarette companies and their ad agencies continue to peddle this vice to you and your kids. Nor do they care if you wind up footing the hundreds of billions of dollars in health care, disability, and long-term care bills that are the direct result of ignoring the dangers of smoking.

Dole made a special point during his days of campaigning of telling a variety of audiences, often in Southern states, that tobacco is not addictive. He proclaimed that while some smokers might find it hard to shake the habit, others do not. Dole also added in these stump disquisitions on the nature of tobacco use that smoking is merely one of a number of things including drinking milk that some people say are not healthy behaviors.

Dole's gonzo views minimizing the addictive and harmful nature of tobacco use were, to put it kindly, incomprehensible, irresponsible, and exceedingly stupid. They were so outrageous that the former surgeon general of the United States, Dr. C. Everett Koop, who is no pantywaisted liberal, wrote and asked Dole why he was wandering around the country proclaiming that tobacco is not addictive since scientific experts, and anybody who smokes heavily, or chews the stuff regularly, knows that it is. Dole's response was to aver that he thinks kids should just say "no" to Joe Camel.

Admittedly, Bob Dole is not running for office any longer. But his legacy on tobacco wheezes on. Indifference to the horrors caused by tobacco is not a stance that any politician or political wannabe should be allowed to adopt. It reeks of hypocrisy.

The fact that tobacco is addictive is not open to debate. Only tobacco-company CEOs and hacks on the dole of the cigarette industry doubt that it is. As published revelations about secret cigarette company memos make abundantly clear, the tobacco industry has been aware for decades that it is in the nicotine delivery and addiction business.

The only way to understand our politicians' inability to speak forthrightly about the addictive nature of tobacco is politics. There is just too much money on the line when it comes to telling the truth about tobacco and its costs.

It is time for for politicians to stop following the lead that Bob Dole set in the last presidential race. It is time for the press to stop accepting obvious dissembling about the dangers of tobacco. The damage done by this addictive substance is simply too overwhelming to ignore. Politicians of all stripes should insist that their party's "big tents" be smoke free.

A Hero In the War On Smoking

In the 1940s the leaders of the then Soviet Union bent science to fit the needs of communist ideology. The government ordered any scientist who said that there was truth in genetics silenced. The only views that would guide agriculture in Russia would be those of Trofim D. Lysenko. Lysenko held that genetics set no limits on what farmers could do to get greater crop yields. This sounded good to totalitarians who wanted to engineer away social and political problems without regard to the limits set by human nature. There was, however, one limit that proved deadly. Lysenko was wrong. By ending funding for all research on genetics and touting Lysenko's nutty theories as true, the communists brought on a famine in the Soviet Union in the 1950s that resulted in the deaths of millions. Your government has a foot on the same path.

Stanton Glantz is a thorn in the side of the tobacco industry. Financed by a three-year grant from the National Cancer Institute he has exposed the role played by lobbyists in manipulating state public health programs supposedly aimed at reducing smoking. For years Glantz and his colleagues at the University of California School of Medicine in San Francisco debunked the cigarette companies' preposterous claims that they did not know about the health dangers of smoking or that nicotine is addictive. Dr. George Lundberg, the editor of the *Journal of the American Medical Association,* calls Glantz one of the "scientists who has done the most important work on tobacco in this decade."

As Glantz began to score points against the tobacco industry, a political campaign was started to shut him up. Articles and letters ran in various right-wing publications and newsletters asking why research inimical to personal freedom (the right to smoke!) was getting federal support.

The blather about individual rights worked. The Appropriations Committee in the House, yielding to enormous pressure from legislators from tobacco-industry states, took the unbelievable step of deleting funding for Glantz's research. There was actually a rider in the appropriation bill $12 billion budget appropriation to the National Cancer Institute explicitly killing off Glantz's $200,000 grant. Like the

Soviet leadership did in the 1950s, Congress is trying to silence someone whose valid scientific findings do not suit their political tastes.

The campaign to silence Stanton Glantz has drawn almost no attention in the mainstream media. It should. Allowing Congress to flack for the tobacco companies by ordering grants terminated is nothing less than political censorship. If you think Congress ought to have the right to recast science in ways more pleasing to its ideological taste, you might want to ask those who lived through the agricultural holocaust of the 1950s in Russia if they think putting politicians in charge of what scientists can study and say is a good idea.

Moral Blarney About Drugs

Old Newt exerted a mighty effort to pin the needle on the goofy meter. The Speaker of the House told an audience in Athens, Georgia, that he favors mass executions for those who supply illegal drugs to the children of our nation. Gingerich defended his somewhat draconian ideas about penal reform by saying he wants to send a message to those who "get rich at the expense of our children that you are signing your own death warrant."

I was impressed by Newt's newfound verve for defending our shores from drug dispensing scumbags but found myself a bit puzzled as to why the Speaker confined his lethal intentions only to those arriving from distant lands to poison our youth. Mr. Gingrich does not have to hang around airports to find those who peddle lethal drugs to kids. All he has to do is pay a visit to those parts of his state and others nearby where tobacco is being grown and made into cigarettes, snuff, and chewing tobacco to find the members of the biggest, best organized, and most lucrative lethal drug-dealing gang in the entire world.

Last year 4,000 people died due to heroin use in this country; 400,000 people died due to tobacco use. The vast majority of those people started using tobacco when they were kids.

As I look out my window right now I can see a group of 14- and 15-year-old girls smoking cigarettes. I am not sure where they bought them but I am certain I know who made them. They are smoking a brand made by Philip Morris, a Richmond, Virginia, tobacco company that has mounted a media barrage to persuade us that their product is just dandy, the company has never done anything to try and hook those who smoke, and that they do all in their power to make sure that only competent adults use it.

Has there ever been such an effusion of moral blarney? Would Newt, you, or I take seriously the same claims if made by the Cali cartel or the Sicilian mob? Yet, our newspapers, radios, and television screens are filled with caterwauling flacks for the tobacco companies bleating about their concern for the health of children, attorneys in fancy suits spewing pap about free choice, and tobacco farmers invoking terms like "family values" and "cultural heritage" to defend the sale of a product that has already killed hundreds of millions of people at a cost of untold trillions of dollars.

Kids are too gullible to fend off the patent nonsense that Philip Morris and other tobacco companies throw at them in the form of slick billboards, sports promotions, and magazine ads. Newt and his pals in Congress are not gullible but the tobacco lobby is powerful. Thus, our politicians find it easier to rant about foreign drug smugglers then protect kids from getting hooked on cigarettes.

Given the level of misery and harm tobacco causes, it ought be viewed with more alarm than heroin and opium. Let's flush those tobacco company CEOs right out of their executive washrooms and round up their lobbyists hanging out at Washington, D.C.'s poshest drinking holes and have them spend a few weeks on death row with their other drug-dealing buddies. Tell them if we find any more kids smoking Newt will hand out the blindfolds. And no one gets a final smoke before Newt tells the firing squad to do its duty.

Should Smokers Adopt?

How rotten are people who smoke? Rotten enough to prohibit them from adopting children?

An adoption agency in Britain has decided to give preference in placing children, especially those under the age of five, to couples who do not smoke. The reasons are simple. Study after study shows that secondhand smoke is bad for babies. More children die of sudden infant death syndrome in households where someone is a heavy smoker. Kids who have parents who smoke are more likely to become addicts themselves.

In checking with adoption agencies in New Jersey, Minnesota, California, and Pennsylvania, none currently disqualify nicotine fiends. Two agencies, one in Pennsylvania and one in Minnesota, did tell me that in open adoptions, where birth mothers meet those who wish to adopt their babies, some moms simply reject anyone who smokes as unacceptable.

I have done a little informal polling on this issue. The first response is almost always that smoking should not be a factor in adoption. But after thinking about it further, my neighbors and colleagues at work almost always change their minds and decide that giving smokers the boot might not be such a bad idea. However, when I ask couples who are trying to adopt or who have adopted children they are unanimous in their view that smoking should be irrelevant. I think the folks who have been down the adoption road are on the right track.

One of the greatest moral revolutions to occur in my lifetime is the change in societal attitudes toward smoking. When I was a kid in the 1960s, smoking was cool. Movie stars smoked. Athletes smoked. My parents smoked. They kept ashtrays around the house. They gave cigarettes to their friends as gifts. The proper moral stance toward smokers was courtesy and consideration. Smoking had nothing to do with sin.

Those days are gone. Smokers, both kids and adults, are now losers. Smoking is not cool. No one keeps an ashtray around their home on the off-chance that an addict might drop by. Giving cartons of cigarettes as presents is ethically akin to giving someone heroin and a needle. Smoking is definitely a sin.

If smokers are irresponsible drug addicts, why let them get their grubby, yellow, nicotine-stained fingers on kids? Because, in fighting the war against tobacco, it is still possible to go to excess.

The problem with banning smokers as parents is that it disqualifies a lot of people who would be great at the task. Sure, it would be better if parents did not smoke. It would also be better if parents did not drive too fast, always used a bath mat, never bought whole milk or lard, had no extramarital affairs, and stopped doing a hundred other things that could hurt their kids.

There are some who will say that letting parents who smoke is to tolerate a vice that is not in the best interests of children. Well, I am all for President Clinton's effort to wage war on tobacco to protect kids. Nothing thrills me more than to see tobacco company executives outed as the hypocrites and liars they are. But vetting prospective parents on the basis of smoking takes the war into places where it should not be fought. It is not clear enough what it takes to be a good parent to throw out those with bad habits. Turning adoption into a race that only the most virtuous can win is neither smart nor fair.

Boobs in New Jersey

Okay, quick, in what state is it easiest to see big boobs on public display? Okay guys, you can stop guessing now about where you think the largest concentrations of strip joints, nude beaches, lap dance emporiums, and video peep-show parlors are. The answer, without question, is New Jersey.

State legislators in the Garden State are making a strong bid to capture and retire the public boob prize. They have managed to do so by finding themselves unable to figure out a way to make it legal for a woman to breast-feed in public.

The need to enact legislation in the Garden State allowing women to bare their breasts to nourish newborns results from a couple of incidents in which women were harassed for nursing in public. In one case a woman was charged with disorderly conduct when she refused to stop breast-feeding her baby while sitting in a food court at a mall. In another, a mom was thrown out of a toy store when the manager told her it was unacceptable for her to be nursing her baby in the aisle.

Incidents like these led to calls to enact a law in New Jersey allowing a woman to nurse in any place in which she has a legal right to be. A law was drafted which also carries a provision that makes sure that breast-feeding is not considered indecent exposure. Sounds simple enough, right? Not when the object of legislative attention is the female breast.

Turns out that some New Jersey legislators find the possibility of a bit of a nursing mother's breast being observed in a public place too much to ask the citizenry to endure. Moreover, the legislators realize that fiendish women bent on exposing themselves in public could hide behind the legalization of breast feeding and indulge their passion for lewd display.

Jersey assemblyman Guy Gregg declared the right to breast-feed anywhere was too expansive. Instead, he argues, stores and restaurants should have the right to insulate the impressionable public from the salacious impact of a baby suckling on a breast. Store owners and businesses ought to be able to send nursing women to private places like the toilet. Another elected guardian of the public's morals, Carol

Murphy, entered the most inane legislative insight of the year contest while explaining her opposition to the proposed law. She told the *Philadelphia Inquirer* "A baby can be used as a weapon to embarrass people. There are women who do exactly that kind of thing."

As a result of insights like these, the bill stalled. The residents of New Jersey remain safe from manipulative exhibitionists who cannot wait to haul babes to malls, parks, and used car dealers so that they can cravenly fling off their blouses and bras, thereby corrupting the morals of an unsuspecting public. There need be no fear from Cape May to Paterson that busty dames will corrupt New Jersey youth with the lame excuse that they were "only feeding the baby." Those who want to see breasts will have to continue to content themselves with the zillions of adult video stores, adult entertainment centers, and strip bars that dot the Jersey landscape.

New Jersey is not alone in its moronic attitudes toward breast-feeding. Only one state, New York, has enacted a law recognizing breast-feeding as a civil right. Every state should do so. Legislators should do everything they can to encourage women to breast-feed. This does not include sending nursing moms to bathrooms, closets, or special rooms. A little public breast-feeding could not hurt. In a society that makes as much money as ours sexualizing women's breasts, it wouldn't hurt to be reminded once in a while that breasts have other functions besides being the object of male ogling.

Corporal Punishment

The little kid was screaming at the top of his lungs. The checkout lines at the supermarket were backed up. Every human being in the greater Philadelphia area in need of 10, 15, or 20 items was standing with or next to me in the optimistically named "express" lanes.

The kid, a boy around six, was hanging on to the cart in front of me. He kept trying to pull it back to the candy rack. His mom, a woman in her late twenties, had an infant in the cart's safety seat. She told her son to stop crying and to quit pulling on the cart. He continued doing both. She yelled at him. My eyes wandered toward the magazine display in the hope that a review of the latest news about alien abductions, Madonna's baby, and JFK Jr. sightings would get me some psychic distance from the child-mother war. The tape ran out in the cash register. The 16-year-old cashier chewed harder on her gum, frowned, and buzzed for the manager. The kid gave the cart another pull. His mother stepped around the cart and slapped him on his behind. Did she do something horribly wrong?

The issue of corporal punishment gets a thorough review in a special issue of *Pediatrics.* Twenty-three experts in children's health, psychology, and human development review what science knows about whether or not parents should hit their kids. Their findings have a lot to say about what happens millions of times each week when adults use hitting or spanking to discipline a child.

In trying to establish whether there is any value to spanking and what harm hitting a child does in the short and long run, the experts restrict their analysis to parental behavior that is intended to deter misbehavior and does not cause physical injury. Blatant violence toward a child is cruel and wrong. It is the mild forms of spanking and slapping that are under review. That is what makes the report so interesting since it is just these forms of discipline which, like the mom at the market, most parents at some time or another, use.

In reviewing the studies that have been done, the experts find that very young infants, under age two, do not understand and cannot be effectively taught by spanking or any form of physical discipline. Studies that followed parents and children over time suggest that aggressiveness and antisocial behavior are more likely to occur when physical punishment is harsher and more frequent. Spanking and other forms of corporal punishment of children who are older than prekindergarten is not effective and may be harmful in the long run. But the experts did find some evidence that the rare spanking of a preschool child may contribute to reinforcing other disciplinary techniques without any apparent harm to the child. Still, noncorporal methods of discipline such as reasoning, positive reinforcement, and "time outs" are always adequate and are the most effective ways to discipline children of all ages.

The conclusions from the experts' review of the scientific data are clear. Getting out the belt or the strap makes no sense and is both a lousy way to parent and unethical. Hitting or spanking an infant or toddler is pointless. The more you hit a child the worse you make things between you and the child in the long run. Spanking, slapping, or hitting may get the attention of a preschooler, as it did that day in the supermarket, but a spank must be used with other nonphysical forms of discipline. If you have ever lost patience and spanked your child, as the mom did in the supermarket, you need not fret about long-term harm but you should know that there are better ways to change bad behavior.

While the rare spanking of a child can get their attention and does not cause long-term harm, rewards, firm instruction, and time-outs do just as well. Corporal punishment has no place in good parenting.

To Die For

Doing the right thing is not easy even when there is a law to guide you. Sometimes, as the basketball career of Nicholas Knapp makes clear, what is right has nothing to do with the law.

On September 19, 1994, Knapp was playing a game of pick-up basketball in his high school gym. Suddenly he collapsed. When the paramedics arrived, Knapp appeared to be dead. The emergency medical technicians managed to get his heart started using CPR and a portable defibrillator. Three weeks later Knapp underwent surgery to put a small defibrillator into his body. This machine will automatically administer a powerful electric shock to Nicholas Knapp's heart should it stop again. It had better work. Knapp wants to start playing Big Ten basketball at Northwestern University in Evanston, Illinois.

Knapp signed a letter of intent to go to Northwestern on November 9, 1994, a month after he had his surgery. Knapp understood that he had a life-threatening cardiac problem, had almost died during a game, and that he had a machine in his belly in case his heart should quit again. He wanted to play ball anyway.

When Knapp showed up on campus in the fall of 1995, the basketball team's head physician, Dr. Howard Sweeney, displayed the first inkling of common sense about the young man's basketball career. He ruled him medically ineligible to play.

Knapp did not lose his scholarship. But he could not practice or play in team games. Knapp loves basketball. He, like 10,000 other guys, thinks he might make it to the pros. So, with the support of his family, he sued Northwestern and its basketball program, alleging discrimination because they would not let him play.

Judge James B. Zagel of the U.S. District Court for the Northern District of Illinois ordered that Knapp be allowed to play. Judge Zagel ruled that basketball was so important to Knapp that he must be allowed to frolic on the hardwood courts in short pants. Not only did Knapp have a legal right to be out there, but Northwestern must provide a defibrillator and a person trained to use it courtside at every practice and game should Knapp's heart show less zeal than Knapp for the rigors of college ball. Perhaps the judge simply forgot to mention that the school ought supply a cooler with a donor heart and a surgeon who knows how to implant it at the ready in case the implantable and the portable defibrillators fail to do the trick.

What was the legal basis that set Knapp free to play roundball? The judge ruled that Section 504 of the Rehabilitation Act of 1973 is Knapp's ticket to hoops. Congress passed the Act to make sure that those with handicaps receive fair treatment at work and school. Judge Zagel gave the Rehab Act a good read and concluded that but for the fact that his heart might fail and kill him, Knapp is as qualified as any other young fellow to rebound for NU.

The judge is wrong. Disability should not count against those who can do a job. But allowing a young man to risk his life to play a game defies common sense. It is not as if Knapp is being kept off the court because he is hearing impaired, has a cleft palate, or is dyslexic. Knapp has a life-threatening medical problem that could kill him. He can live without basketball.

Nicholas Knapp wants to play. He wants to play badly enough that he is willing to risk his life. The law has taken Knapp's side. But it is the wrong side to take. There is a difference between forbidding discrimination and the need to protect kids against bad decisions.

Drunk Driving

Joseph Duvall is 28 years old. If you get anywhere near Louisiana he might kill you. Joseph Duvall is a repeat drunk driver.

The Denham Springs, Louisiana, man spent part of last year in Parish Prison when he was arrested for driving while intoxicated. The arrest came less than a year after Duvall spent three months in jail on an earlier DWI conviction. Altogether Duvall has been arrested seven times for DWI. When Louisiana state troopers hauled Duvall in last June, he had a valid driver's license even though under state law it should long since have been revoked.

When arrested, Duvall refused to take a breath test, sobriety test, or answer any questions put to him by the cops. When his case comes to a trial it will be the troopers' word against his that he was drunk when arrested. Assistant District Attorney Kim Landrum has been down this road before with repeat drunk-driving offenders: "It is going to be a hard row to hoe," she admits, to keep Joe off the road.

Some chronic drunk drivers encounter things other than the cops while motoring. Keith Brian Tracy, a 32-year-old Wind Gap, Pennsylvania, man, was sentenced to 24 to 36 months in prison for killing Leona Kerwin when his car smashed into her as he made a left turn while driving drunk at what police say is a dangerous intersection. It was his third drunk-driving conviction.

Our national inability to get tough on drunk driving has led some employers and insurance companies to look for ways to avoid paying the bills. Companies in Texas, Colorado, and Arkansas have said their insurance plans will not pay for any medical care necessary as a result of drunk-driving accidents. Insurance companies such as Blue Cross of Maryland periodically ask state legislators to allow them to turn down medical bills submitted by persons and their families injured or paralyzed as a result of driving while drunk.

Ducking the crushing costs of drunk driving by throwing people with broken bones and crushed spinal columns out of the hospital is not the best way to solve this problem. Hospitals are not going to throw paraplegics into the street. If companies are allowed to exempt drunk-driving accidents from their insurance plans, you and I will wind up paying through Medicaid or Medicare for the care of the Joe Duvalls, Keith Tracys, and their victims once they go broke.

Companies are also pretty selective about what counts as a hospital bill they do not like. Smash yourself and your kin to bits while drunk and driving and you are off the health plan. But no problem if you are willing to risk bodily harm picking up heavy crates, inhaling noxious chemicals, operating dangerous machinery, or storing toxic substances. Somehow the sins your employer deems worthy of dumping off the health plan are less troubling if the sin helps somebody make a buck.

The solution to drunk driving does not lie in playing hot potato with the bill. The solution required is sobriety tests, mandatory jail time, tougher treatment programs, loss of license for repeat offenders, and confiscation of car, boat, snowmobile, or motorcycle for anyone convicted more than three times of DWI. If we don't get tough you will continue to face the loss of both your health and your savings every time someone gets loaded and gets behind a wheel.

Medical Marijuana

Imagine you are dying and in a great deal of pain. There is a drug available that can safely relieve your pain, but your doctor cannot prescribe it. The drug has been used since 1840 and is known to be extremely effective. Still, it is against the law to to prescribe the drug. Marijuana is the drug, laws making it illegal to use for medical purposes ought to be changed.

For almost a decade the Drug Enforcement Administration has refused to follow the advice of its own legal counsel and permit doctors to prescribe marijuana. You do not have to be someone who, unlike the president, actually inhaled, to understand that it makes no sense to prohibit the use of marijuana for the relief of pain. Lester Grinspoon and James Bakalar, a physician at the Harvard Medical School and a lawyer specializing in drug policy argue that the ban makes no sense.

The case against allowing doctors to prescribe marijuana rests on three points. First, legalization will undercut society's efforts to fight drug abuse. Second, synthetic alternatives to marijuana are available so there is no need to let anyone smoke dope legally. And last, there is no reliable scientific evidence that marijuana really can do what its proponents claim—relieve cramps, migraine, and most important, help control the symptoms of nausea caused by chemotherapy and other treatments for cancer and AIDS. None of these arguments can hold up under scrutiny.

There is no reason whatsoever to think that allowing doctors to prescribe marijuana to terminally or seriously ill patients will turn kids into drug addicts. The sight of someone ravaged by cancer smoking a joint in a hospice is not likely to inspire any teenager to head out onto the street to cop a couple of blunts.

True, a form of synthetic marijuana has been available in capsule form since 1985. Physicians can and do prescribe it. But it does not have the same effect on every patient. Some find smoking easier and more effective than swallowing pills. Does it make any sense to insist that someone in pain must use a synthetic, more expensive but possibly less effective version of a substance that they could grow in their backyard?

The argument that more proof of efficacy is needed might make sense if marijuana was a new, poorly understood drug of dubious safety. But marijuana has been around longer than aspirin. If you are dying, its risks and harms are zero.

It is time to bring reefer madness to an end. Doctors ought to have the right to prescribe marijuana for those who are terminally ill or imminently dying. The feds should heed the pleas of the citizens of Arizona and California who have legalized the drug for the terminally ill. Let the dying do what they must in order to make dying bearable.

Olestra

The food police are on the loose again. They are moaning and groaning about the decision of the Food and Drug Administration to allow a fat substitute, Olestra, on supermarket shelves. They cannot stop yammering about innocent fatties leveled by stomach cramps and nutrients being vacuumed out of overfed innards if this stuff is put in our foods. These critics do not know what they are talking about. They are all thin.

Fat-free foods in our chips and fries means a lot to us porkier people. No longer will we face the torture of standing as a bloated object of scorn and derision when seen by our neighbor sneaking tastes out of packages at the snack food display at the local GrandVon's AcmePiggleUnion. Small children will no longer ask if they can stand under the overhang of our guts in the parking lot and play while we empty our treasure of blubber-inducing products into the back of our sport-utility vehicles. In a couple of months we will be able to stand proudly next to you in the checkout line whipping jumbo-sized bags of crunchy or gooey sin out of our carts without having the checkout girl and the bag boy exchange knowing mooing sounds. Rush Limbaugh will be able to buy a Speedo.

Science, however, unlike the food police is not perfect. Olestra, which Procter & Gamble (its makers), hope to slip into your snacks in order to permit you to gobble down potato chips and wolf down fries with abandon, does admittedly come with a price tag. Olestra will not be easy for everyone to swallow. It is a price the tubby among us must ask themselves if they are willing to pay. Am I so addicted to grease that I am willing to endure cramps, diarrhea, and the risk of having most of the vitamins that somehow manage to get into my body leached right out again as the phony fat molecules ply their way through my intestines?

The food fascists think my answer and yours should be no. The most vociferous are the folks at the Center for Science in the Public Interest. They are beside themselves that the FDA has decided to turn the other cheek so to speak to Olestra. They think that a body without vitamins in it is too high a price to pay for the chance to eat as much ripples and dip as you like.

It must be noted that those now grumbling about fat substitutes are the very same people who allege that a Mexican dinner consisting of tacos with mountains of cheese, refried beans, and a large cola is not good for you. No one is going to listen to this sort of obvious disinformation. I have seen many people eat prolifically at Mexican fast-food restaurants and not expire from cardiac arrest until they were home and in bed.

There are other food do-gooders around as well. Many of them have degrees in nutrition. They note that simply substituting for fat in our foods will make us eat more foods that are of no value.

Let me note for the record that nutritionists are the same people who provide the food served in hospitals and high school cafeterias. What more need I say? Anyway the burly among us who think a food pyramid is some obscure Egyptian fast-food joint are not likely to have had a lot of vitamins and leafy green veggies in their diet to begin with. Letting a fat substitute into cookies, chips, ice cream, and fries will not alter the larger man and woman's vitamin equation, since negative numbers cannot be used in the measurement of vitamins.

Americans change their diets—never. The blimpiest among us must be left free to maintain hoglike food habits just as long as our gastrointestinal problems do not interfere with the liberty of others. It is the American way. Split a bag of fat-free chips with me Rush?

Cholesterol Fever

This nation has lost its marbles when it comes to staying healthy. No, I am not talking about the proclamation by the leadership in the House and Senate that there will be no more picking on tobacco companies on Capitol Hill. I refer to a recent announcement by Dr. Harlan M. Krumholz and a prestigious team of Yale University cardiologists and statisticians that high cholesterol levels are not predictive of heart disease in people in their late seventies and older.

This announcement was greeted with a sigh of relief all around the country. Newspapers, radio, and television blared forth the happy news that great-grandma could again eat bacon and eggs for breakfast. But is this a message that requires scientific confirmation in order to be persuasive? Is there no age at which the health police deem it appropriate to shift from prevention to indulgence?

The reprieve from dietary purgatory for those in their advanced golden years was issued on the basis of a four-year study that followed 997 men and women whose average age was 79. The researchers, who announced their findings in the November 2, 1996, issue of the *Journal of the American Medical Association,* found no correlation between high cholesterol levels and an increased risk of heart attack.

Some medical experts were not so impressed by the Yale findings. More data are needed before we can be absolutely sure that high cholesterol does not put octogenarians at greater risk of death they harrumphed.

What is going on here? Can it really be true that people in their late seventies and eighties are desperately trying to control their diets and take drugs to prevent heart disease? Is there no age at which doctors, drug companies, dietitians, and nutritionists will raise the white flag in the battle against the clogged artery? Is the obsession to live forever so pervasive that we actually have to spend your tax dollars to prove that it is just fine to let people past their eighth decade ingest doughnuts without anxiety?

The pursuit of health has gone so far off the deep end that we consider it newsworthy to report that it is difficult to prevent death among 80-year-olds. We are a nation that has spawned a phalanx of highly paid health professionals who will not rest until scientific studies establish beyond any shadow of a doubt that high cholesterol at age 85 does not pose an obstacle to having your name read on your one-hundredth birthday by Willard Scott on the *Today Show.*

Do we really need statistically significant data to persuade ourselves that it is not sinful to eat butter, steak, and ice cream without guilt when you reach the age when Bob Dole impresses you as a spry young gallant? Is there no age bracket for whom we are willing to accept the idea that quality of life is more important than quantity?

Look, I believe older Americans have as much right as the rest of us to the finest care the medical system of this nation has to offer, including hanging around office waiting rooms engaged in the remedial reading of *Highlights for Children* while listening to Lite music hits from the 1970s. But a society that permits its oldest members to spend their days fretting about cholesterol lest they die prematurely is a society that might want to recheck its compass on the subject of health prevention.

Even if we could all stave off a heart attack at age 85 by forswearing pizza and hot dogs at 80, something else is going to get us. No matter how many fat dissolvers you scarf down, no matter how many points you knock off your lipid count by ingesting mass quantities of fiber, if you are a lot more than a decade past your first Social Security check, the Grim Reaper is about ready to finish arguing with you. My advice is invite him over for a big slice of cake and ice cream on your eightieth birthday and see if you can at least distract him a bit longer by bringing up the subject of his cholesterol count.

Health Nuts

Having a nice time enjoying your summer vacation? There are plenty of people who think you shouldn't. Health Puritanism is running amok across the land.

The new Puritanism acquired its strength through victory in the long-overdue war on smoking, and the anxieties of a graying baby-boom generation who are slowly realizing they are mortal. A gaggle of health zealots is taking full advantage of the culture's collective neurosis about aging and death by extending their priggishness to every nook and cranny in your daily life.

Hardly a day goes by without a warning souring what used to be a fun activity. Going to the shore? Forget it, the sun will kill you. Ready for dinner? Not if there is anything with a hue other than green on your plate or it could be your last meal. Want to watch some television? The programs will rot your brain, the electrical emissions will mutate your offspring, and the couch you sit in might as well be decorated with a headstone.

To my astonishment, a physician has actually published a paper in which he takes direct aim at health fanaticism. His message is just what the doctor ordered as an antidote to those dedicated to driving us bonkers about risks and dangers to our health. The doctor wants you to have fun!

Dr. James McCormick, Professor of Community Health and General Practice at Trinity College in Dublin, Ireland, issued his call to sanity in the respected British medical journal, *The Lancet*. Does the good doctor urge us all to quaff yet another glass of celery juice or add still one more mile to our dreary morning jog? No, he does not. The doctor writes that the members of his profession "would do better to encourage people to live lives of modified hedonism, so that they may enjoy, to the full, the only life that they are likely to have."

Yup, those of you who just gagged on your morning bacon or who cannot stop this page from jumping around before your eyes because you are already on your fourth cup of coffee, read the doctor's advice correctly. He said the aim of medicine should not be to try and figure out how best to hector you about marginal risks and remote dangers. It should, instead, be to encourage you to have fun in moderation.

The mob making a living as health Cassandras will not take a liking to Dr. McCormick's counsel. It does not square with their litany of anxiety-provoking, hyperventilating, and just plain scary pronouncements about whatever it is that might maim, mutilate, disable, disadvantage, impair, or annihilate you.

Think about the warnings you are expected to absorb in any given month. Vitamins will kill you. The ozone can't protect you. The air is poisonous. Caffeine will deform your babies. Sperm counts are falling and no one knows why. There are additives in your milk that will cause you to grow a tail. Bran won't save you unless you wear the box on your head to cushion the impact of the high volume of malicious, fast-moving celestial matter that is pointed straight at your noggin from all points in the galaxy. Cancer of the stomach, uterus, pancreas, liver, and breast is inevitable unless you drink seven quarts of spring water a day. Even if you turn yourself into a human fire hydrant, you are only delaying the inevitable fatal fall in your bathroom, stabbing by a coworker, or stroke, aneurysm, or cardiac arrest of unknown origin. One might arrive at the opinion that the roles once played in our culture by abstract ideas of hell, limbo, and eternal damnation have found secular expression in the abstract ideas of high blood pressure, bad cholesterol, and ideal weight.

McCormick's call for sanity in matters of health is rooted in solid scientific evidence. The benefits of a healthy lifestyle can be gotten as readily, he notes, from a life full of moderation as one of fanaticism.

The goal of health promotion is not health. It is to produce health so that you can enjoy a happier life. If health promotion is not fun, it is not worth it. Obsessing about your health is no way to live. Scaring others about small risks and dangers to their health is no way to make a living.

Cyberporn

Over the past few weeks I did something I almost never do in my office. No wise guy, it wasn't work. I locked my door. I had decided to take a visit to the redlight districts of the Internet to see for myself what sort of pornography is out there. I did not want anyone waltzing into my office to find the ethics professor staring hard at the nether regions of some lewd image.

A study in the Georgetown University *Law Journal* by Matthew Rimm, a student at Carnegie Mellon University, set me in pursuit of dirty pictures. Rimm claims cyberspace is awash in filth. He says more than 900,000 dirty pictures are floating around where little kids can easily find them. There are, he warns, also a wide variety of discussion groups full of lascivious dialogue, perverted topics, and kinky gab.

The media lost its collective mind when confronted with a mix of sex and computers. *Time* put Rimm's study on its cover. TV talk shows have been parading an unending horde of alleged victims of computer sex. Editorial writers who cannot tell hard drive from hard core fulminated about filth on the net. Nipping at their heels is a pack of overheating members of Congress. Senators Charles Grassley of Iowa and James Exon of Nebraska put on their best Elmer Gantry faces to wave copies of *Time* around on the Senate floor demanding censorship of smut on the net.

Next in line for apoplexy were the free speech computer nerds. When Congress began breathing hard over finding sex in electronic space, free speech computer wonks set out to discredit Rimm and his study. They say it is nuts to claim that the net is awash in naked bodies.

I decided to see for myself. I began by wandering through various websites and discussion groups looking for sex. Pretty tame. I could have found more racy images by turning on an aerobics class on ESPN2.

Maybe I did not know where to look. I called on some of my more computer savvy friends to help me wend my way to CyberSodom.

Soon, I found what I was looking for. There are dirty pictures, in fact, a few absolutely filthy ones, out there.

Sex magazines like *Playboy, Hustler, and Penthouse* have sites with pictures you can view. A lot of places charge you to see dirty pictures. Nearly all have warnings that those under 21 should stay away.

Smut is on the net. But although some of what is there is raunchy and surely unfit for kids, it is, oddly, not sexy. Current computer graphics are not anywhere close to providing the lewd imagery you can get on your cable TV or a glossy magazine. The chat groups are not as lewd as what can be heard on the zillions of 900 "adult" numbers that show up on late night TV and clog the back pages of many newspapers and magazines.

Cyberspace certainly has less sex on it than you can find at the average newsstand or movie rental store. Rather then censor the Internet, Congress might want to have the ATF and FBI stake out the top drawer of dad's bureau—who knows what the kids might find in there under the socks!

Safety First

Are you lying down as you read this? You should be. You are about to read something you will hardly ever find in your newspaper— good news. Really. Yes, it is news that even a hardened cynic like you will have to admit is good. Okay, okay I will also tell you some worrisome stuff if you read this to the end. But, hey, don't complain. You could be reading somebody else's column about Bosnia, the national debt, or AIDS and you know they aren't going to tantalize you with any rays of hope in those bleak precincts.

Do you think more Americans died in accidents in 1969 or in 1994? Hint: there are lots more people alive in the United States today than there were 25 years ago. 1994? Wrong. You really are a cynic. Remember, I promised you good news.

Twenty one percent fewer people died from accidents in 1994 than in 1969. Statistics from the National Safety Council say that 116,385 people died in car accidents, motorcycle crashes, fires, falls, or in workplace mishaps in 1969. In 1994, 92,200 people died from these same causes. In 1969 accidental death was the fourth leading cause of death for all Americans. In 1996 it moved back to fifth place.

So why the good news? The answer is simple. Public and private regulations and laws aimed at increasing safety worked. By mandating safety belts in our cars, safety glasses in the workplace, smoke detectors in our homes, national minimum age laws for drinking alcoholic beverages, insisting on tougher penalties for drunk driving, and tightening mandatory safety standards for our appliances, trucks, tools, clothes, and toys, a real dent has been made in the tragic accidents that are a major source of death and disability.

Not only has the push for safety saved lives, it has saved money. Accidents accounted for more than $400 billion in lost income and medical expenses last year, but that sum would have been much, much higher had the rate of accidental death not taken such a huge dip.

It is simply incredible that benefits of an increased emphasis on safety though law, regulation, and private initiatives have gone more or less unnoticed in the media. But safety goggles and smoke detectors are not especially wondrous pieces of technology. And their impact on our health is hard to determine since the benefits of low-cost, preventive technology is only apparent in trends over many, many years.

Now for the bit of bad news. One group of your fellow citizens, Congress, are peculiarly indifferent to the saving of lives and the reduction of costs brought about by the increased emphasis in federal laws on safety in the home, highways and the workplace. The current Congress has assigned itself the goal of dismantling the very laws and regulations that have saved tens of thousands of lives and hundreds of billions of dollars.

Congress is especially keen on abolishing speed limits and helmet laws. It wants to deregulate safety in the trucking industry. It believes that the only safe place for an FDA official or an OSHA inspector is the unemployment line.

Politicians might lie but statistics don't. You are much less likely than your parents were to be hurt or killed in an accident at home, at work, or while traveling. That is good news that even your congressional representative should be able to appreciate.